Sex and Control

Monographs in German History

The complexities and peculiarities of German history present challenges on various levels, not least on that of historiography. This series offers a platform for historians who, in response to the challenges, produce important and stimulating contributions to the various debates that take place within the discipline.

For full volume listing, please see pages 184 and 185

Sex and Control

Venereal Disease, Colonial Physicians, and Indigenous Agency in German Colonialism, 1884–1914

Daniel J. Walther

berghahn
NEW YORK • OXFORD
www.berghahnbooks.com

Published in 2015 by
Berghahn Books
www.berghahnbooks.com

Library of Congress Cataloging-in-Publication Data

Walther, Daniel Joseph, 1965- , author.
Sex and control : venereal disease, colonial physicians, and indigenous agency in German colonialism, 1884-1914 / Daniel J. Walther.
p. ; cm. -- (Monographs in German history ; volume 36)
Includes bibliographical references and index.
ISBN 978-1-78238-591-2 (hardback) -- ISBN 978-1-78238-592-9 (ebook)
I. Title. II. Series: Monographs in German history ; v. 36.
[DNLM: 1. Sexually Transmitted Diseases--Germany. 2. Colonialism--history--Germany. 3. History, 19th Century--Germany. 4. History, 20th Century--Germany. 5. Physician's Role--history--Germany. 6. Sexual Behavior--history--Germany. WC 140]
RA644.V4
616.95'100943--dc23

2014033536

British Library Cataloguing in Publication Data
A catalogue record for this book is available from the British Library

Printed on acid-free paper.

ISBN 978-1-78238-591-2 hardback
ISBN 978-1-78238-592-9 ebook

To Linda, for your unflagging support and patience.

Contents

ACKNOWLEDGMENTS

There are a number of people and organizations I would like to thank for making this project possible—more than I can fully remember. To start, I'd like to begin by recognizing those people who have played essential roles in shaping this book, either directly or indirectly. At the top of the list is my good friend and colleague, Staffan Müller-Wille, who read earlier versions of these chapters and pushed me to be more precise and more compelling in my prose and arguments. Indeed, without his input, the completion of the manuscript would have taken considerably longer and the book would have suffered. Of course, I want to thank Veronika Lipphardt and the other members of her Independent Research Group at the Max Planck Institute for the History of Science, or MPIWG (Berlin, Germany). Either directly or indirectly, her remarks and the comments of others helped shape this book through feedback on the paper I shared with them or in other conversations—too many, in fact, to recount them all. I'm also extremely grateful to Veronika and the MPIWG for inviting me to be a part of her group, "Twentieth Century Histories of Knowledge About Human Variation," for it enabled me to present my findings and interact with others, as well to have the time, space, and resources to conduct research and write. During my time there, I made considerable progress on this project, which helped expedite the writing process after I returned home. A debt of gratitude also goes out to Axel Hüntelmann, Cornelie Usborne, and my good friend Matthew Fitzpatrick, all of whom provided useful comments, suggestions, and questions along the way.

In addition, the outside reviewers and editors of the various publications that provided foundational material for the manuscript contributed significantly to sharpening my analysis and prose. Specifically, I want to thank Matthew Kuefler at the *Journal for the History of Sexuality*; Graham Mooney at the *Social History of Medicine*; the former editor of the *German Studies Review,* Diethelm Prowe; and Nina Berman, Klaus Mühlhahn, and Patrice Nganang, editors of a collection on African and Asian responses to German colonialism.

I also want to thank my colleagues at Wartburg College, in particular Terry Lindell and Erika Lindgren. Even though our scholarly interests are decidedly different, their camaraderie, encouragement, and support provided an environment where I could be productive.

A special thanks goes to the staff at the Max Planck Institute, especially those working in the library. They make the life of a researcher collecting materials appear almost effortless. Further, the staff at the various archives I visited—i.e., the National Archives of Australia, the Bundesarchiv Lichterfelde, and the Military Archive in Freiburg—was always ready to assist me in finding and obtaining the documents essential for my research.

Of course, this project would not have been possible without financial support. Both the Academic Exchange Service (DAAD) and the Fulbright Kommission (Germany) made it possible for me to spend considerable time in Germany carrying out the necessary research. Also, Wartburg College's Faculty Development Committee and the Office of the Vice-President for Academic Affairs provided additional funding for my trips to Germany and Australia and granted me a year-long sabbatical in 2011–2012.

Moreover, I am greatly appreciative of the support I received from the people at Berghahn Books, especially my editors Adam Capitanio and Elizabeth Berg, who guided me throughout the publication process and made it a smooth experience.

Finally, I want to thank my family for their patience, understanding, and support while I worked on this project. Their love gave me inspiration and the drive to finish the project, especially during those moments when my enthusiasm for it was waning.

Earlier versions of material appearing in this book was originally published in the following:

"Sex, Public Health and Colonial Control: The Campaign Against Venereal Diseases in Germany's Possessions, 1884–1914," *Social History of Medicine* 26, no. 2 (2013): 182–203. Reprinted with permission from Oxford University Press.

"Sex, Race, and Empire: White Male Sexuality and the 'Other' in Germany's Colonies," *German Studies Review* 33, no. 1 (February 2010): 45–72. Reprinted with permission from Johns Hopkins University Press.

"Sex and Control in Germany's Overseas Possessions: Venereal Disease and Indigenous Agency," in *German Colonialism Revisited: African, Asian and Oceanic,* eds. Nina Berman, Klaus Mühlhahn, and Patrice Nganang (Ann Arbor: The University of Michigan Press, 2014). Reprinted with permission by the University of Michigan Press.

"Racializing Sex: Same-Sex Relations, German Colonial Authority, and Deutschtum," *Journal of the History of Sexuality* 17, no.1 (2008): 11–24. Reprinted with permission by the University of Texas Press.

Abbreviations

AA	German Foreign Office (*Auswärtiges Amt*)
AkG	*Arbeiten aus dem kaiserlichen Gesundheitsamte*
ASTH	*Archiv für Schiffs- und Tropenhygiene*
BArch	German Federal Archive—Lichterfelde (Bundesarchiv)
BArch-MA	German Federal Archive—Military Department Freiburg
DKG	German Colonial Society (Deutsche Kolonialgesellschaft)
DNG	German New Guinea (Deutsch-Neuguinea)
DOA	German East Africa (Deutsch-Ostafrika)
DSWA	German Southwest Africa (Deutsch-Südwestafrika)
MB	*Medizinal-Berichte über die Deutschen Schutzgebiete*
NAA	National Archives of Australia
RKA	Reichskolonialamt (Imperial Colonial Office)
VD	Venereal disease(s)

INTRODUCTION

Sex and its regulation occupied a central position in the German colonial enterprise; they permeated the political, social, economic, and cultural life of the colonies. As various scholars have already demonstrated,[1] formal sexual relationships between the races and the progeny from such encounters challenged the colonial order and the future of the colonies as German possessions, while responses to these threats strengthened the gender and racial hierarchy by banning mix marriages and relegating offspring to a lower racial status. The aim of these policies was not to prevent sexual relations between whites and non-Europeans. Rather, they attempted to redirect white male sexual desire. Thus, as concubinage and miscegenation over time became less of an acceptable option for European men, the only real publicly permissible alternatives were either marrying German women or engaging a prostitute.

However, due to the demographics of the colonial situation, there were always too few white women, while indigenous women were in abundance. Consequently, for many white men, the only real choice was turning to a prostitute for their sexual gratification. Prostitution, though, was closely associated with venereal diseases (VD), and according to colonial health authorities, VD not only weakened military effectiveness and economic vitality—two cornerstones of German colonialism—but also white rule itself, the very foundation of the colonial enterprise. Indeed, venereal diseases posed not only an immediate danger, but also one to the future because they ostensibly prevented the reproduction of the African, Asian, and Pacific Islander labor force and, more importantly, the white race.

Notes for this section begin on page 8.

As in Germany, physicians as public health officials were charged with combatting this perceived danger to the colonial endeavor. Further, like their colleagues at home, to prevent the spread of VD, or at least mitigate the effects of dissemination, doctors used both normative and surveillance measures based on scientific knowledge and bourgeois perceptions of health and race. Their primary goal, though, was to transform targeted populations into supporters of good public hygiene, and hence advocates for the colonial order. Nonetheless, physicians also employed surveillance measures. In fact, over time they increasingly resorted to more punitive actions in order to curb the spread of venereal diseases.

Due to the racial hierarchy in the colonies, doctors could require more bodies to submit to medical supervision than was possible in Germany. At home, medical officials could only exercise moderate authority over the bodies of prostitutes and, to a lesser degree, over enlisted military personnel. In the colonies, medical authorities not only required medical examinations of prostitutes and soldiers (both European and non-European), but also of those indigenous groups perceived to be essential to the colonial order or threatening that order. Moreover, unlike the situation in Germany, they introduced policies and facilities to enforce compliance with medical diagnoses and treatments, which included the confinement of those who attempted to leave before they were healed. In Germany, physicians would only achieve greater authority with the passage of the 1927 Law for Combatting Venereal Diseases. Later, under the Nazis, their power would surpass that exercised in the colonies.[2]

In pursuing normative and surveillance measures to fight VD, doctors provided colonial officials with another means to try to regulate and change the lives of non-Europeans that was not directly political. Rather, medical discourses were employed to justify various actions that ultimately contributed to broadening colonial rule. The objective was to eliminate or reduce the threat of venereal diseases through education, regulation, and coercion. Such polices were necessary to ensure the territories had a viable military force, a productive labor pool, and a healthy white population—all deemed essential for the maintenance and perpetuation of German colonialism.

Unlike most studies of German colonialism that focus on more obvious forms of disciplinary power, such as the use of military or police force,[3] this book takes a biopolitical and comparative approach to the study of German colonialism through the lens of discourses surrounding health. The concept of biopolitics, introduced by Michel Foucault,[4] refers to the ways in which the state and its agents exercised power through governmental practice for the purpose of regulating both individual bodies and entire populations. Biopolitical practices cover a wide range of techniques and targets, but typically took an indirect approach rather than working through straightforward disciplinary intervention, such as in the regulation of sexual behavior achieved through the propagation of scientific knowledge and discourses of "sexuality." Because the health of the population was increasingly seen as a fit and proper target of government policy, such biopolitics were also productive as much as repressive, aimed at both "knowing" a population as novel objects of knowledge and policy and steering individuals, as "subjects," in directions that benefited the state as well as themselves—indeed, actively recruiting them into this process of medico-moral government. In the case of doctors in Germany, the aim, as elsewhere, was to replace the outmoded understandings and unsanitary practices of the working classes with modern, scientific knowledge and rational behavior, instilling in them the values of health, productivity, and morality.[5]

This medical modernization process became part of European imperialism in the nineteenth and twentieth centuries. Specifically, it required supplanting indigenous views and comportment with these middle-class values. According to the scholar David Arnold, this meant that "medicine and public health … formed part of the hegemonic project of the colonial regime, a project aimed at promoting the security and legitimacy of colonial rule, and, concurrently, at eliminating or subordinating all rival systems of authority."[6] Yet, as Megan Vaughan has demonstrated in her study of illness in Africa, the subjectification of Africans was a complicated phenomenon and was often more ideal than realized. Yes, some colonial subjects were "produced," but most remained "objects" and the focus of surveillance. In other words, the system was not primarily "productive," but, according to Vaughan, rather "repressive" like the situation in early modern Europe.[7]

However, I would contend that the "repression" that took place in the colonies within the context of the struggle against VD as a result of noncompliance with public health measures was not necessarily a throwback to the early modern period. Rather, it was modern because the focus, the means, and the rationale had changed. The primary focus was on disciplining the population through surveillance and normalization. Modern medicine sought to transform society and define who belonged in the nation-state and who did not according to the authority of scientific knowledge. The mechanisms for achieving this conformity and responding to incidents of noncompliance relied primarily on medical discourses of health and disease that shaped educational, legislative, and surveillance measures that focused on individuals' bodies and population groups. Under the auspices of protecting the common, greater good and with a didactic purpose intended to shape appropriate comportment, those that did not comply with such measures were removed until they no longer posed a threat to the community.[8]

This was certainly the case during the campaign to stop the spread of venereal diseases in Germany's colonies. Doctors did share their knowledge of VD and public hygiene in an effort to replace indigenous knowledge and attitudes through their medical discourses and practices, but the ongoing spread of the disease resulted in them resorting to increasingly more surveillance and punitive activities in order to achieve their goals and to correct disobedient behavior. Consequently, this book enables us to gain insights into the less obvious ways Germans tried to exert authority in the colonial situation, including the extent of colonial power and the limitations of it.

Because of its focus on medicine, this book also highlights the role of modernity in German colonialism. Of course, there were strong antimodern tendencies in the German experience, but as several scholars have pointed out, the modern was also present. However, most researchers interpret the colonies as places where modern ideas were tested, the so-called laboratories of the modernity.[9] This book, though, explores the *application* of the modern in the colonial context. The colonies were primarily locations where doctors applied their knowledge and understanding, not where they tested them. Admittedly, doctors did test new medicines and treatments on colonial subjects. Further, the colonial environment did impact the policies they pursued. But, the colonial setting did not change physicians' core beliefs and goals. In both settings, doctors continued to believe in science and that, ultimately, scientific knowledge would prevail. Moreover, because of their faith in scientific medicine, the end justified the means. This did not mean that the colonial setting did not influence the policies they pursued and how they interacted with targeted populations. Quite the contrary, they had to adapt to the colonial environment. Further, because they were not in Germany, they did not face many of the restrictions their colleagues there encountered, at least not with regards to non-European policies. Thus, in the overseas territories, they implemented the policies they did because they could, which in the end went beyond what was possible at home.

Works do exist that examine colonial medicine, but these are limited in number and focus.[10] The majority concentrate on the history of medicine in the colonial environment, and therefore do not contribute much to our understanding of German colonialism. One exception is Wolfgang Eckart's *Medizin und Kolonialimperialismus,*[11] which provides a detailed narrative of the medical actions pursued in Germany's colonies and offers a useful explanation for the motivation of colonial physicians. However, it misses the full extent of how colonial physicians conceived of themselves and their role in the colonies.

As Ann Stoler has argued, "colonial cultures were never direct translations of European society planted in the colonies, but unique cultural configurations, homespun creations in which European food, dress, housing, and morality were given new political meanings in the particular social order of colonial rule."[12] This also applied to the realm of public health and the campaign to fight VD. Due to the colonial setting, doctors were able to go beyond what their colleagues at home could do. Consequently, this book sheds light on what was "shared' and what "differed"[13] between the center (Germany) and the periphery (the colonies), and thus provides additional insights into the tensions that existed between original intensions and colonial realities.

In large part, a significant difference between the two was the racial component, which was invoked not only to justify physicians' actions, but also to account for the ongoing threat posed by VD. Indeed, much to the frustration of these doctors, the success of their measures depended largely on the decisions and behavior of nonelite indigenes targeted by these programs. Some autochthons did not comply with German regulatory requirements for prostitutes; compulsory health examinations for indigenous laborers, soldiers, the wives of soldiers, and prostitutes; enforced medical treatments for those found infected;

and educational programs. Their tactics and motivations varied, but collectively their nonviolent, nonconfrontational actions contributed to limiting the success of these various measures aimed at reducing the spread of venereal diseases, at least according to German health officials. Simultaneously, some indigenes did willingly register as prostitutes, allowed themselves to be examined for VD, underwent treatment until cured, and heeded the health advice shared by German colonial physicians. Like those who did not conform to German expectations, they had their own motivations, but nonetheless they did contribute in part to the success of these measures.

In both types of responses, their actions did not necessarily need to be viewed exclusively as either resistance to or compliance with German requirements and expectations. Rather, those who took a particular action also did so in accordance with their own agenda.[14] As the works of James Scott[15] and Detlev Peukert[16] have shown, opposition to a hegemonic power manifested itself in a wide array of often apparently insignificant ways. Obviously, outright resistance did take place in the colonial setting. However, there were also actions taken that were often nonviolent and individualistic, usually amounting to nonconformity and not outright opposition or resistance. And even if there was an act of outright protest, it may not have been directed at the colonial system per se, but rather at a particular policy or action on the part of the authorities. However, when viewed collectively, these individual acts had a substantial impact on the colonial enterprise and revealed the degree to which the objects of control accepted or rejected the values being imposed upon them by colonial authorities. According to Scott, "whatever the response [of the colonized], we must not miss the fact that [their] action[s] … changed or narrowed the policy options available to the state." He called these acts "*everyday forms of resistance.*"[17]

However, it is extremely difficult to access the voices of indigenous commoners, individuals who often had direct contact with colonial authorities, and hence had numerous opportunities to be influenced by them and to shape colonial policy. Generally speaking, historical documents that directly record their experiences often do not exist. Rather, their lives and experiences are recorded in the writings of others, often their colonial rulers. As Subaltern Studies has demonstrated, it is possible to discern "fragments" or "traces" of suppressed narratives, i.e., the stories of the subaltern, in the records of colonial officials.[18] These voices can often be found in the slippages that occur in the application of colonial authority and the responses to them.[19] Thus, in the case of German public health policies, in particular the fight against the spread of venereal diseases, the actions and behavior of indigenous commoners is found in the reports and essays of German colonial physicians.

Such an approach facilitates, therefore, a deeper understanding of the colonial situation from the perspective of the colonized. Specifically, insights are gained on the practices employed by everyday Africans, Asians, and Pacific Islanders in response to the German public health measures to stop the spread of venereal diseases, how their actions caused colonial authorities to adapt their approaches to combating this health concern, and ultimately how their behavior impacted the efficacy of these measures. Moreover, by looking at the sources in this manner, a glimpse into the motivations of the various actors is achieved.

Overwhelmingly, the literature on indigenous responses to German colonialism explores the more obvious forms of opposition, namely armed and collective. Moreover, those that do explore individual actors tend to focus on male elites.[20] These approaches are readily apparent in the burgeoning historiography of the Nama and Herero Wars in German Southwest Africa.[21] Thus, most do not examine the everyday encounters of commoners with their colonial interlopers. Eckert does do this to a degree in his *Grundbesitz, Landkonflikte und kolonialer Wandel,* but ultimately he also focuses on male elites within society.[22] In one case study, Philipp Prein does investigate nonviolent opposition to German colonialism in Southwest Africa, yet he concentrates on collective action and not individual acts that had a cumulative effect.[23]

Few studies exist that address similarities and differences across the German colonies (pancoloniality). The most notable exception is George Steinmetz's book,[24] which demonstrates how precolonial perceptions of non-European peoples and the socioeconomic background of colonial officials resulted in different "native" policies in Qingdao, Samoa, and Southwest Africa. This book, however, shows that perceptions of non-Europeans from a medical perspective were largely uniform. Further, the responses to this medical threat were nearly the same throughout the overseas territories. The main variation was in which groups were targeted, which in turn was often determined by the extent of colonial control.

In addition, venereal diseases were not unique to German experience, but rather were prevalent in other imperial powers' colonies. As Philippa Levine[25] and Philip Howell[26] have demonstrated, VD also constituted a threat to and influenced the nature of British imperialism. Thus, the fight against venereal diseases was part of a larger European phenomenon. Indeed, in her recent dissertation, Deborah Neill successfully argued that the activities of German and French doctors in Cameroon were part of European modernization.[27]

Consequently, this book situates the German fight against venereal diseases within the larger context of European imperialism. Specifically, it points out commonalities and divergences between German and British colonialism. Many of the more general conclusions regarding sex, race, and prostitution are similar to those of Levine and Howell. However, in terms of specifics, the German experience differed from the British. For example, British efforts focused on prostitutes and military personnel, while in the German case attention was given to those associated with economic productivity and white rule in addition to military power and prostitution.

The book begins with a chapter describing the situation in Germany and then is divided into three main sections. This first chapter, "Doctors, Prostitution, and Venereal Disease in Germany," explores the role of physicians as public health officials within the context of industrialization and urbanization. It focuses especially on the role of prostitution in German society and its challenges to bourgeois values and public health because of its association with venereal diseases. It concludes with doctors' responses to this threat, which included the medicalization of German society that allowed for the objectification of the lower classes and efforts to subjectify them. Objectification justified the necessity for specific policies that were intended to reduce the perceived threat and that could also lead to the subjectification of targeted populations.

The second chapter, "Male Colonial Sexuality," examines the perceptions of male sexuality in the colonial situation, colonial sexual demographics, types of sexual contact, and colonial sexual politics. The latter attempted to address the challenges to bourgeois values and colonial rule through mixed marriage bans in some of the colonies, while still providing men with access to acceptable forms of sex. Due to demographics, this meant primarily non-European women through prostitution, which is the focus of the third chapter ("Prostitution in Germany's Colonies"). This chapter explains in detail the growth of prostitution in each territory, the different types of prostitution, and the various reasons for its expansion during the colonial period, including why women engaged in it.

In part 2, chapter 4, "The Threat of Venereal Disease," explores the hazard VD posed to the strength of colonial armies, the vitality of the labor force, and the health of the white, ruling population. The next chapter, "Assessing the Threat Statistically," provides a detailed statistical analysis of venereal diseases in the colonies and the role of statistics in promoting the colonial order of race and health and proper comportment. Chapter 6, "Racial Categories, Venereal Disease, and the Colonial Order," examines how the category of "race" in the statistics was defined through medical discourses and used to objectify Africans, Pacific Islanders, and Asians in order to justify the various policies pursued.

In part 3, chapter 7, "Preventative Measures," explains the various educational efforts doctors directed at targeted populations with the goal of turning them into willing participants in the fight against VD (i.e., their subjectification). These efforts were directed primarily at colonial soldiers (both European and non-European) and indigenes. The next chapter, "Disciplining the Body," explores the various surveillance measures used to identify the infected. Unlike the situation in Germany and the British colonies, medical supervision in Germany's possession included a broader spectrum of the colonial population, including not just prostitutes and military personnel (both European and non-European), but also other non-European female and male groups connected to the economy and white rule. The racial hierarchy and the medical "othering" of these different groups made this possible. Chapter 9, "Treating the Body," focuses on medical treatments as a form of surveillance by ensuring that infected individuals did not contaminate healthy bodies. It also examines how the indigenous body became a site for medical experimentation and the limits of medical knowledge. The last chapter in this section, "Assesseing the Surveillance," assesses the impact of these different policies. I begin with an evaluation of what was accomplished and how, and conclude with an explanation of the limitations of the policies and why. A discussion of indigenous agency runs throughout the chapter as well as an exploration of the more normative measures employed in response to African, Asian, and Pacific Islander actions. Indeed, these populations had a direct impact on the methods German doctors used in the colonies, often causing them to adjust some policies to encourage more indigenes to seek medical treatment or to pursue more punitive measures that served to ensure immediate compliance and to educate the infected that noncompliance was inappropriate behavior.

Notes

1. Katharina Walgenbach, "Rassenpolitik und Geschlecht in Deutsch-Südwestafrika (1907–1914)," in *Rassenmischehen—Mischlinge—Rassentrennung. Zur Politik der Rasse im deutschen Kolonialreich,* ed. Franz Becker (Stuttgart: Steiner Verlag, 2004), 165–183; Birthe Kundrus, "'Weiß und herrlich': Überlegungen zu einer Geschlechtergeschichte des Kolonialismus," in *Projektionen. Rassismus und Sexismus in der Visuellen Kultur,* ed. Annegret Friedrich et al. (Marburg: Jonas Verlag, 1997), 41–50; Fatima El-Tayeb, "Verbotene Begegnungen—unmögliche Existenzen. Afrikanisch-deutsche Beziehungen und Afro-Deutsche im Spannungsfeld von *race* and *gender,*" in *Die (koloniale) Begegnung. AfrikanerInnen in Deutschland 1880–1945. Deutsche in Afrika 1880–1918,* ed. Marianne Bechhaus-Gerst and Reinhard Klein-Arendt (Frankfurt: Peter Lang, 2005), 85–95; Katharina Walgenbach, *"Die weisse Frau als Trägerin deutscher Kultur": Koloniale Diskurse über Geschlecht, "Rasse" und Klasse im Kaiserreich* (Frankfurt: Campus, 2005).
2. Lutz Sauerteig, *Krankheit, Sexualität, Gesellschaft. Geschlechtskrankheiten und Gesundheitspolitik in Deutschland im 19. und früheren 20. Jahrhundert* (Stuttgart: Franz Steiner Verlag, 1999), 428–435; Michael Burleigh and Wolfgang Wippermann, *The Racial State: Germany 1933–1945* (New York: Cambridge University Press, 1991); Robert Proctor, *Racial Hygiene: Medicine under the Nazis* (Cambridge, MA: Harvard University Press, 1988).
3. For example, Horst Drechsler, *Let Us Die Fighting: The Struggle of the Herero and the Name Against German Imperialism (1884–1915*), 3rd ed. (Berlin: Akademie Verlag, 1980); Jürgen Zimmerer, *Deutsche Herrschaft über Afrikaner. Staatlicher Machtanspruch und Wirklichkeit im kolonialen Namibia* (Münster: Lit, 2002); Trutz von Trotha, *Koloniale Herrschaft: zur soziologischen Theorie der Staatsentstehung am Beispiel des "Schutzgebietes Togo"* (Tübingen: J.C.B. Mohr, 1994); Walter Nuhn, *Kamerun unter dem Kaiseradler: Geschichte der Erwerbung und Erschliessung des ehemaligen deutschen Schutzgebietes Kamerun: ein Beitrag zur deutschen Kolonialgeschichte* (Dessau: Wilhelm Herbst, 2000).
4. For example, see Michel Foucault, *The History of Sexuality: An Introduction* (New York: Vintage Books, 1990); and Foucault, *The Archaeology of Knowledge* (New York: Pantheon Books, 1972); and Foucault, *The Birth of Biopolitics: Lectures at the Collège de France. 1978–1979,* ed. Michel Senellart (Houndsmill, NH: Palgrave Macmillan, 2008). For a more thorough discussion of Foucault's concept of "productive power," see Hubert Dreyfus and Paul Rabinow, *Michel Foucault: Beyond Structuralism and Hermeneutics* (Brighton: Harvester Press, 1982), 126–182. Megan Vaughan provides a good overview of Foucault's position within the context of colonialism in *Curing Their Ills: Colonial Power and African Illnesses* (Stanford, CA: Stanford University Press, 1991), 8–12.
5. Ute Frevert, "Professional Medicine and the Working Classes in Imperial Germany," *Journal of Contemporary History* 20 (1985): 644.

6. David Arnold, "Public Health and Public Power: Medicine and Hegemony in colonial India," in *Contesting Colonial Hegemony: State and Society in Africa and India,* ed. Dagmar Engels and Shula Marks (London: British Academic Press, 1994), 131–151, 140.
7. Vaughan, *Curing Their Ills,* 10–19. For an example of this early modern repression, see Isabel Hull, *Sexuality, State, and Civil Society in Germany, 1700–1815* (Ithaca, NY: Cornell University Press, 1996).
8. Michel Foucault, *Discipline and Punish: The Birth of the Prison* (New York: Pantheon Books, 1977), especially 184. Though Paul Weindling does not explicitly refer to this as a modern phenomenon, his discussion of health and race in late nineteenth- and twentieth-century Germany suggests a similar conclusion. Paul Weindling, *Health, Race and German Politics between National Unification and Nazism, 1870–1945* (Cambridge: Cambridge University Press, 1989).
9. Dirk van Laak, "Kolonien als 'Laboratorien der Moderne'?" in *Das Kaiserreich transnational: Deutschland in der Welt 1871–1914,* ed. Sebastian Conrad and Jürgen Osterhammel (Göttingen: Vandenhoeck & Ruprecht, 2004), 257–279. For examples, see also Klaus Mühlhahn, *Herrschaft und Widerstand in der "Musterkolonie" Kiautschou: Interaktionen zwischen China und Deutschland 1897–1914* (Munich: Oldenbourg, 2000); Harry Rudin, *Germans in the Cameroons 1884–1914: A Case Study in Modern Imperialism* (New Haven, CT: Yale University Press, 1938).
10. Margit Davies, *Public Health and Colonialism: The Case of German New Guinea 1884–1914* (Wiesbaden: Harrassowitz Verlag, 2002); Hiroyuki Isobe, *Medizin und Kolonialismus: Die Bekämpfung der Schlafkrankheit in den deutschen "Schutzgebieten" vor dem Ersten Weltkrieg* (Berlin: Lit Verlag, 2009).
11. Wolfgang Eckart, *Medizin und Kolonialimperialismus Deutschland 1884–1945* (Paderborn: Ferdinand Schönigh, 1997).
12. Ann Stoler, "Rethinking Colonial Categories: European Communities and the Boundaries of Rule," *Comparative Studies in Society and History* 31 (1989): 136–137.
13. Sebastian Conrad uses the terms "shared" and "divided," but "different" seems more appropriate. Conrad, *Globalisation and the Nation in Imperial Germany* (Cambridge: Cambridge University Press, 2010), 5. See also Conrad and Shalini Randeria, "Geteilte Geschichten: Europa in einer postkolonialen Welt," in *Jenseits des Eurozentrismus: Postkoloniale Perspektiven in den Geschichts- und Kulturwissenschaften,* ed. Conrad and Randeria (Frankfurt: Campus, 2002), 9–49; Shalini Randeria, "Geteilte Geschichte und verwobene Moderne," in *Zukunftsentwürfe: Ideen für eine Kultur der Veränderung,* ed. Jörn Rüsen, Hanna Leitgab, and Norbert Jegelka (Frankfurt: Campus, 2000), 87–96.
14. Andreas Eckert, *Die Duala und die Kolonialmächte: Eine Untersuchung zu Widerstand, Protest und Protonationalismus in Kamerun vor dem Zweiten Weltkrieg* (Münster: Lit, 1991), 8.
15. James Scott, *Weapons of the Weak: Everyday Forms of Peasant Resistance* (New Haven, CT: Yale University Press, 1985).
16. Detlev Peukert, *Inside Nazi Germany: Conformity, Opposition, and Racism in Everyday Life* (New Haven, CT: Yale University Press, 1987).
17. Scott, *Weapons of the Weak,* 36.
18. For example, Gyanendra Pandey, "Voices from the Edge: The Struggle to Write Subaltern Histories," in *Mapping Subaltern Studies and the Postcolonial,* ed. Vinayak Chaturvedi (London: Verso, 2000), 281–299.
19. For instance, Ilan Kapoor, *The Postcolonial Politics of Development* (Oxon: Routledge, 2008).
20. For example, John Iliffe, *Tanganyika under German Rule, 1905–1912* (London: Cambridge University Press, 1969); Peter Hempenstall, *Pacific Islanders under German Rule: A Study in the Meaning of Colonial Resistance* (Canberra: Australian National University Press, 1978); Peter Hempenstall and Noel Rutherford, *Protest and Dissent in the Colonial Pacific* (Suva: Institute of Pacific Studies of the University of the South Pacific, 1984); Eckert, *Die Duala und die Kolonialmächte.*

21. For example, Gesine Krüger, *Kriegsbewältigung und Geschichtsbewußtsein: Realität, Deutung und Verarbeitung des deutschen Kolonialkrieges in Namibia 1904 bis 1907* (Göttingen: Vandenhoeck and Ruprecht, 1999); Jürgen Zimmerer and Joachim Zeller, eds., *Genocide in German South-West Africa: the Colonial War (1904–1908) in Namibia and its Aftermath* (Monmouth, Wales: Merlin Press, 2008); Andreas Bühler, *Der Namaaufstand gegen die deutsche Kolonialherrschaft in Namibia von 1904 bis 1913* (Frankfurt: IKO, Verlag für Interkulturelle Kommunikation, 2003).
22. Andreas Eckert, *Grundbesitz, Landkonflikte und kolonialer Wandel: Douala 1880 bis 1960* (Stuttgart: Franz Steiner, 1999).
23. Philipp Prein, "Guns and Top Hats: African Resistance in German South West Africa, 1907–1915," *Journal of Southern African Studies* 20, no. 1 (March 1994): 99–121.
24. George Steinmetz, *The Devil's Handwriting: Precoloniality and the German Colonial State in Qingdao, Samoa, and Southwest Africa* (Chicago: University of Chicago Press, 2007).
25. Philippa Levine, *Prostitution, Race and Politics: Policing Venereal Disease in the British Empire* (New York: Routledge, 2003).
26. Philip Howell, *Geographies of Regulation: Policing Prostitution in nineteenth-century Britain and the Empire* (Cambridge: Cambridge University Press, 2009).
27. Deborah Neill, "Transnationalism in the Colonies: Cooperation, Rivalry, and Race in German and French Tropical Medicine," PhD dissertation (University of Toronto, 2005).

PART I

Male Sexuality and Prostitution in the Overseas Territories

Chapter 1

Doctors, Prostitution, and Venereal Disease in Germany

*B*y the last decades of the nineteenth century and in the early years of the twentieth, venereal diseases appeared to be on the rise in Germany. According to hospital records, between 1877 and 1909 the number of cases for gonorrhea had risen by 182 percent and for syphilis by 19 percent throughout the German Empire. Despite contemporary criticisms of the statistics, there was nonetheless a general consensus among experts that VD appeared to be on the rise. In fact, some physicians even argued that the figures were probably higher. This rise was accompanied by an increase in prostitution. Though prostitution had been around for centuries, industrialization led to an apparent rise in prostitution. Estimates at the turn of the century ranged between 100,000 and 200,000 prostitutes active in Germany; by 1914, it was believed that about 330,000 prostitutes worked in the country.[1]

Politicians, moralists, and public health officials viewed both VD and prostitution as symptoms of the moral decline of German society that undermined the physical and cultural vitality of the nation.[2] This degeneration was most visible in urban centers, which were perceived as harboring "the germs not only of crime and epidemic diseases such as typhus and cholera, but also of venereal infection and immorality."[3] In particular, VD was seen as endangering the nation's military strength, productivity, and ability to reproduce. Because the values of the nation had become synonymous with those of the middle classes during the empire,[4] the bourgeoisie perceived this situation as signs of the "impending crisis of the family, a decline in moral standards, and the resulting threat to the stability of"

Notes for this section begin on page 20.

middle-class values.[5] These included the ideals of "hard work, competition, [and] achievement," but above all hard work and the productivity associated with it.[6]

Consequently, the health of the nation was intimately linked to the ability of the population to be productive and to reproduce itself.[7] "The central problem of public health ..., the connection between the health of the general population (*Allgemeinheit*) and the health of the individual (*des einzelnen*), can be explained through the productive capacity of the work of the entire society or through individual threats."[8] Already in 1873, Max von Pettenkofer was one of the first to calculate how much the wealth of a German city could be increased if the health of the population was improved. Further, in the age of nationalism, this also included the ability of the nation to defend itself from competitors and to expand.[9]

Consequently, any threats to the productivity of the nation or its ability to propagate itself had to be met, dangers closely tied to ideas of evolution and degeneration. Beginning in the later nineteenth century, theories of evolution and degeneration were intertwined in efforts to promote the development and perpetuation of the nation and simultaneously to combat the various threats to the strength and continued vitality of the state. Thus, evolution was closely linked to the ideas of production and reproduction, while degeneration was connected to those factors that endangered these concepts.[10]

In the last decades of the nineteenth century, these threats emanated primarily in urban locations among the working poor. Indeed, cities and the people that inhabited them became associated with the rise in tuberculosis, venereal diseases, and alcoholism.[11] "The poor population, which live under substandard health conditions, or certain general life influences ... threaten as contagious pollutants the function and reproduction of the social body."[12]

In order to deal with these problems, the functions, powers, and personnel in government at the local, state, and eventually national level expanded. Consequently, new career opportunities for professionals opened up not just in engineering, building, finance, and law, but also in medicine. These new openings enabled physicians to use their professional knowledge in service to the state, either directly or indirectly. Thus, though a free profession, their rise to prominence was intimately tied to the expansion of state power.[13]

Doctors believed that through their scientific education they could "reorder society" for the advancement of humanity. Indeed, they argued that only they possessed the requisite knowledge essential for this task.[14] Repeatedly physicians asserted that they worked for "the advancement of science," which would ultimately "improve the wellbeing of humanity."[15] Advances made in germ theory were notable examples of this. Not only did germ theory promise "to uncover the microscopic origins of many diseases, [it] also contributed to a growing confidence that western science was the answer to many of the world's social ills."[16]

Initially doctors and the state responded to this threat by using public health "to discipline and restrain the industrial workforce." Such a punitive approach utilized "a system of medical police with powers to quarantine, disinfect and, in the case of certain contagious diseases and mental illnesses, to detain in custody in hospital."[17]

But, as the nineteenth century began to close, many of these threats were increasingly seen not as problems of morality, but rather as medical and social problems that could "be solved by public health policy."[18] From the perspective of physicians, scientific knowledge could be applied "to such diverse problems as disease, waste, climate control, entomology, urbanism, architecture, clothing, agriculture, and public hygiene."[19] Increasingly, then, German society was medicalized,[20] especially after the state began utilizing such knowledge and individuals with expertise in these areas.

This focus on the health of the nation "allowed the medical profession to claim a leading role in imposing bourgeois values onto the rest of the" country,[21] and thus simultaneously promote evolutionary policies and combat degenerative practices. As members of both the bourgeoisie and the medical profession, their objective now became to "civilize" the masses in the ideals of the modern state, i.e., the middle-class values of rationality, productivity, and health.[22] The working class needed to be educated in what constituted a healthy, "orderly, self-disciplined and sober lifestyle." Health would be used to achieve "a cohesive and integrated society during the upheavals of industrialization,"[23] albeit one based upon bourgeois values. In other words, the working classes would be subjectified, thereby becoming active agents in promoting middle-class values of health and prosperity. Although the working class increasingly identified with bourgeois values,[24] coercive measures, however, were not entirely abandoned.

In order to justify their actions, physicians and other members of the middle class first objectified the lower classes as a threat to the current social and political order. They did this by ascribing specific traits or attributes to all members of this group that were in opposition to bourgeois norms, and hence turned them into an "other."[25] From their perspective, the working class was "short-sighted, selfish, [and] sectional."[26] Further, it was unaware of good health practices and correct sexual comportment. Hence, its behavior challenged middle-class norms of production and reproduction. Such a perspective not only legitimized the bourgeois status quo, it also justified middle-class efforts to interfere in the lives of the lower classes. "At times, such programs of intervention were inspired by philanthropy."[27]

Thus, physicians used medical knowledge, and the power that increasingly accompanied it, especially after the introduction of health insurance, to shape the behavior of the lower classes in their campaign to "civilize" them. One concrete way doctors tried to do this was by joining or establishing various middle-class organizations. Some of these organizations included the Association for Social Policy (*Verein für Sozialpolitik*), the German Association for Poor Relief and Charity (*Deutscher Verein für Armenpflege und Wohltätigkeit*), and the German Society for Combating Venereal Disease (*Deutsche Gesellschaft zur Bekämpfung der Geschlechtskrankheiten,* or DGBG). Physicians often constituted an important block or assumed influential positions within these groups. This was particularly apparent in the DGBG. The primary goal of these societies was to preserve middle-class ideals by combating the threats to them, which often included improving the living conditions of the lower classes and instilling in them bourgeois ideals.[28]

In addition, many doctors utilized their expertise and knowledge to serve the state either directly or indirectly. For instance, those that worked for the state became "more and more specialists responsible for public health, especially for the prevention and fight against infectious diseases (*übertragbarere Krankheiten*)."[29] They were aided by advances in medical science, which enabled doctors to more effectively diagnose and treat more diseases with the passage of each year. This affirmed their belief that they could reorder the world, even though they ignored the fact that many diseases during the time remained uncured or that their treatments were often extremely painful.[30] This also applied to the understanding and treatment of venereal diseases.

Along with the vice unit of the police (*Sittenpolizei*), university-trained doctors played a significant role in the struggle to respond to the spread of VD and immorality. Although there was no required registration requirement for venereal-infected individuals during the Second Empire, the state attempted to exercise a degree of control over those segments of the population that it could ostensibly more easily regulate. These included primarily military personnel and prostitutes.

Because of the hierarchal nature of the armed services and their importance to the German nation, military physicians could and did subject soldiers and sailors to medical supervision. A great deal of effort went into subjectifying enlisted men, many of whom belonged to the objectified lower-middle and lower classes. On a regular basis, doctors provided these men with "educational lectures and brochures [that] warned … [them] of the dangers of extramarital sexual relations" in an effort to influence their behavior. They also gave them prophylactics and instructed them in their proper use.[31] As a precaution, and perhaps out of recognition that the comportment of these men could not be changed immediately (or even at all), doctors conducted regular medical screenings of armed service personnel, which included a VD examination.[32] In the Prussian army and the imperial navy, those who did not register themselves to be disinfected after becoming infected with VD would be punished. Those infected, though, had to leave their anonymity behind and report to the sanitation personnel. Only then would they be required "to admit [this] unwanted, but in the military tolerated, offense against the moral norms" and undergo treatment. As the medical historian Lutz Sauerteig noted, many soldiers unsurprisingly did not submit to the supervised disinfection.[33]

Nevertheless, there were limits on what the military high command could do. It was not until World War I that a registration (*Meldepflicht*) for VD-infected soldiers and a concomitant forced treatment was even deemed politically feasible. Depending on the location and the state of origin of the military unit—e.g., Bavarian—such registrations were either voluntary or required or nonexistent. Even before the war, the emperor prohibited in 1912 the sale of prophylaxes and the installation of machines dispensing them in the barracks. This was in response to pressure from various morality organizations that saw these automats undermining the morals of young soldiers and sailors.[34]

In German society, though, most efforts went into monitoring prostitutes. The 1871 criminal code did not make prostitution itself illegal. Its existence was deemed essential as a "safety-valve" for male sexuality. According to contemporary thinking, even though men, due to their rational ability, were supposed to be able to control their sexual drive, they still needed an outlet for their sexual needs. Prior to marriage men could satisfy themselves through prostitution, while ultimately heterosexual marriage was supposed to provide men with a more respectable means to achieve sexual gratification as well as contribute to the stability and growth of the state. Even in such formalized relations, though, it was still acceptable for men to seek satisfaction outside of marriage if their needs were not being met. Moreover, according to contemporary attitudes, prostitution was preferable to other forms of sexual gratification, such as masturbation or same-sex relations. The latter two undermined bourgeois notions of health, reproduction, and masculinity.[35] Thus, in the late nineteenth and early twentieth centuries "the dominant paradigm for sexuality [was] overwhelmingly male and heterosexual" and bourgeois.[36]

However, despite the important function prostitutes provided to many middle-class men, they were marginalized from the bourgeois world. The body of the prostitute was seen as the "representative sexualized female body" and "a site of abnormal indulgence." Moreover, as part of this supposed pathological behavior, the "body of the prostitute [also] came to be … synonymous with venereal disease." According to the scholar Mary Spongberg, "the terms 'social disease,' referring to syphilis and gonorrhea, and 'social evil,' referring to prostitutes, came to be used interchangeably. Prostitutes were seen as both physically and morally responsible for the spread of venereal disease. They were seen not merely as agents of transmission but as inherently diseased, if not the disease itself." The consequence of this was that the body of the prostitute became medicalized. Her body was a place "where disease could and did fester,"[37] and hence necessitated and justified supervision by physicians.

This perspective remained even after the health insurance reforms of 1903 transformed prostitution and VD from a moral problem into a medical and social concern. Indeed, "medical men clung tenaciously to the idea of the prostitute's body as an infectious site and attempted to maintain control of this body, in spite of their increased knowledge regarding the aetiology of the disease and their growing power to cure it." The prostitute's diseased body still threatened the health of the body politic.[38]

Due to her medical and sexual marginalization, the prostitute became the "easiest target for sexual regulation."[39] The 1871 national law enabled police to "arrest and subject to a medical examination anyone suspected of being a prostitute." Moreover, it criminalized procuration.[40] The new law also outlawed bordellos, though Hamburg continued to use this system. Most cities resorted to the system of *Kasernierung* (or "quartering"). In general, this system required prostitutes to register "in their place of residence," "issued [them] … an identification book," "required [them] to undergo frequent medical examinations, … and admitted [them] to [a] hospital if they had contracted an infectious disease."[41] The main goal of these measures was "the total disciplining and subordination of prostitutes,"[42] or more specifically their bodies.

It was, however, impossible to regulate all prostitutes, especially in the urban areas. First, near the end of the nineteenth and at the beginning of the twentieth centuries, the nature of prostitution changed. Due to social and economic conditions among the laboring classes, many women turned to prostitution. However, for many it was not a profession, but rather a response to "insecure, poorly paid" and seasonal employment. Thus, prostitution became a "temporary solution" to difficult economic situations. Consequently, during this time, most prostitutes were occasional or situational (*Gelegenheitsprostituierte*), not professional ones (*Gewerbs-* or *Berufsprostituierte*).[43] Second, local governments lacked sufficient personnel to register every prostitute, especially if more and more of them engaged in occasional or opportunity prostitution. "The regulation system in Germany failed to ensnare … every prostitute in the cities, where the strength of the morals police in manpower terms was hopelessly inadequate."[44]

Not until 1927 did health officials gain a powerful legal tool in their efforts to fight VD and to regulate infectious bodies. The 1927 Law for Combatting Venereal Diseases required anyone infected with a venereal disease to undergo mandatory treatment by a university-trained physician. Thus, both prostitutes and now their customers were subject to medical supervision. Those who did not complete their treatment or continued to have sexual intercourse while still infected were reported and doctors could commit them to a lock hospital.[45]

Nevertheless, major discoveries in the field of bacteriology assisted physicians in the campaign to fight VD. For example, in 1879, the German Alfred Neisser identified the bacterium that caused gonorrhea (*gonococcus*). Ten years later, an Italian, Augusto Ducrey, discovered the pathogen for ulcus molle or chancroid. This enabled a differentiation to be made between the primary effects of syphilis and ulcus molle, and hence which disease afflicted an infected individual. Not until 1905 did Fritz Schaudinn and Erich Hoffman determine the source of syphilis (*Treponema pallidum,* or Treponema S). By 1910, various scientists had identified three additional types of nonsexually transmitted *Treponema*: Treponema Y, the cause of yaws; Treponema C, the agent that caused pinta; and Treponema M, or endemic syphilis. One year after the discovery of Treponema S, August Wassermann developed a serological test for syphilis, the so-called Wasserman test. However, it was not always dependable, for it had a tendency to produce false positives for other diseases or someone already treated for the disease or to produce no reaction for an individual infected with syphilis.[46]

Nonetheless, physicians used this scientific knowledge "to segregate the unfit and socially deviant" from the fit.[47] As the nineteenth century ended and the twentieth began, the medically unfit became diseased objects whose afflictions needed to be diagnosed and treated. Patients were no longer individuals, but rather primarily objects of medical inquiry. According to feminist theory, the person as object meant the lack of agency, individuality, autonomy, history, and personality. Moreover, the object became "a tool for the objectifier's purposes." Quite often the object was identified with her/his body.[48] Or, quite simply, patients had become a "thing" (*Ding*)[49] that doctors examined and treated for the advancement of medical science and the well-being of society. Essentially, their treatment became a scientific or technical problem and their identity was reduced to a statistic.[50]

The most visible representation of the objectified patient was in fact the statistic. The collection of data accompanied the rise of modern states, for through statistics the complexity of society could be simplified by reducing populations to types. This knowledge, including the typologies produced, enabled those in positions of authority to try to appropriate, regulate, control, and manipulate populations.[51]

Already in the early years of the German Empire, those interested in public health recognized the importance of medical statistics. Part of the impetus to establish the Imperial Health Office (*kaiserliches Gesundheitsamt*) in 1873 was to collect data on a national level that would provide insights into the health of the nation after industrialization and urbanization had brought significant changes to the political and social order in Germany. According to Axel Hüntelmann, "The medical statistic was considered a central element of public hygiene."[52]

Ultimately, then, the diseased and lower classes were both objectified, albeit in two different ways. The objectification of the diseased focused on an individual, reducing that person to an entity without agency that could be acted upon by the medical profession as it saw fit. Meanwhile, the objectification of the lower classes entailed the assignment to them of a behavior that threatened bourgeois norms. Therefore, steps had to be taken to reduce or eliminate this challenge. It was diseased prostitutes who embodied both forms of objectification. Consequently, because of their behavior they needed to be liminalized from mainstream society, which included regular medical examinations so that the diseased body could be identified and treated before it could reenter society.

In the colonial setting, doctors would utilize similar methods to combat the spread of venereal disease. As in Germany, VD was seen as a threat to political and social order in the overseas possessions. Though charged with maintaining the health of the European population and ensuring economic productivity, male—especially white—sexual behavior exacerbated the health situation in the colonies. Miscegenation, cohabitation, and the progeny from interracial relationships threatened to undermine the future of German colonial rule. Increasingly then, the only sanctioned forms of sexual relations for white men were either marriage to a European woman or prostitution. But, because of demographics, the most viable option was prostitution. However, as in Germany, prostitution brought with it increased risks of venereal infection. In responding to this challenge, colonial physicians objectified the threatening populations, and in the process contributed to maintaining the colonial order based on middle-class ideals, which now included a racial hierarchy with middle-class, heterosexual whites at the top.

Notes

1. Sauerteig, *Krankheit, Sexualität, Gesellschaft*, 68–88; Andrea Jenders and Andreas Müller, *"Nur die Dummen sind eingeschrieben ..." Dortmunder Dirnen- und Sittengeschichte zwischen 1870 und 1927* (Dortmund: Geschichtswerkstatt Dortmund: 1993), 93; Lynn Abrams, "Prostitutes in Imperial Germany, 1870–1918: Working Girls or Social Outcasts?" in *The German Underworld: Deviants and Outcasts in German History*, ed. Richard Evans (London: Routledge, 1988), 189; Richard Evans, "Prostitution, State and Society in Imperial Germany," *Past and Present* 70 (1976): 108.
2. Lutz Sauerteig, "'The Fatherland is in Danger, Save the Fatherland!' Venereal Disease, Sexuality and Gender in Imperial and Weimar Germany," in *Sex, Sin and Suffering: Venereal Disease and European Society*, ed. Richard Davidson and Lesley Hall (London: Routledge, 2001), 77, 79. See also Christiana Hilpert-Fröhlich, *"Auf zum Kampfe wider die Unzucht." Prostitution and Sittlichkeitsbewegung in Essen 1890–1914* (Bochum: SWI-Verlag, 1991), 7; Jenders and Müller, *"Nur die Dummen sind eingeschrieben,"* 93; Regina Schulte, *Sperrbezirke. Tugendhaftigkeit and Prostitution in der bürgerlichen Welt* (Frankfurt: Syndikat, 1979), 7.
3. Rudi Bleys, *The Geography of Perversion: Male-to-male Sexual Behaviour outside the West and the Ethnographic Imagination, 1750–1918* (New York: New York University Press, 1995), 151.
4. Sauerteig, "'The Fatherland is in Danger,'" 77; Karl-Heinz Leven, *Die Geschichte der Infektionskrankheiten: Von der Antike bis ins 20. Jahrhundert* (Landsberg and Lech: Ecomed, 1997), 116; George Mosse, *Nationalism and Sexuality: Respectability and Abnormal Sexuality in Modern Europe* (New York: Howard Fertig, 1985), 16; Daniel Walther, "Racializing Sex: Same-Sex Relations, German Colonial Authority, and Deutschtum," *Journal of the History of Sexuality* 17, no.1 (January 2008): 23–24; and David Blackbourn, "The German Bourgeoisie: An Introduction," in *The German Bourgeoisie: Essays on the Social History of the German Middle Class from the late eighteenth to the early twentieth Century*, ed. David Blackbourn and Richard Evans (London: Routledge, 1991), 9.
5. Abrams, "Prostitutes in Imperial Germany," 189.
6. Blackbourn, "The German bourgeoisie," 9–10. See also Richard Evans, "Family and Class in the Hamburg Grand Bourgeoisie, 1815–1914," in *The German Bourgeoisie,* 130; Weindling, "Bourgeois Values, Doctors and the State: The Professionalization of Medicine in Germany 1848–1933," in *The German Bourgeoisie,* 199.
7. Paul Weindling, "Hygienepolitik als sozialintegrative Strategie im späten Deutschen Kaiserreich," in *Medizinische Deutungsmacht im sozialen Wandel des 19. und 20. Jahrhunderts,* ed. Alfons Labisch and Reinhard Spree (Bonn: Psychiatrie-Verlag, 1989), 37–38.
8. Gerd Göckenjan, *Kurien und Staat machen: Gesundheit und Medizin in der bürgerlichen Welt* (Frankfurt: Suhrkamp, 1985), 131.
9. Henry Sigerist, *Civilization and Disease* (Ithaca, NY: Cornell University Press, 1945), 61–62; Weindling, "Bourgeois Values, Doctors and the State," 218.
10. Nancy Stepan, "Biological Degeneration: Races and Proper Places," in *Degeneration: The Dark Side of Progress,* ed. J. Edward Chamberlin and Sander Gilman (New York: Columbia University Press, 1985), 97–120; George Mosse, *Toward the Final Solution: A History of European Racism* (New York: Howard Fertig, 1985 [1978]), 82; and Daniel Kevles, *In the Name of Eugenics:*

Genetics and the Uses of Human Heredity (New York: Alfred Knopf, 1985), 70–84, 180–182). See also Bleys, *The Geography of Perversion,* 145–146, 156, 160.

11. Weindling, *Health, Race and German Politics,* 190.
12. Göckenjan, *Kurien und Staat machen,* 131.
13. John Breuilly, "Urbanization and Social Transformation, 1800–1914," in *Germany: A New Social and Economic History,* vol. 3, *Since 1800,* ed. Scheilagh Ogilvie and Richard Overy (London: Arnold, 2003), 208; Weindling, "Bourgeois Values, Doctors and the State," 198–223.
14. Neill, "Transnationalism in the Colonies," 108; Gerd Göckenjan, "Wandlungen im Selbstbild des Arztes seit dem 19. Jahrhundert," in *Medizinische Deutungsmacht,* 89–102, specifically 91–93; Paul Weindling, "Bourgeois Values, Doctors and the State," 199; Lutz Sauerteig, "Salvarsan und der 'ärztliche Polizeistaat': Syphilistherapie im Streit zwischen Ärzten, pharmazeutischer Industrie, Gesundheitsverwaltung und Naturheilverbänden (1910–1927)," in *Medizinische Bewegungen im Deutschen Reich (ca. 1870–ca. 1933),* ed. Martin Dinges (Stuttgart: Franz Steiner Verlag, 1996), 193.
15. Barbara Elkeles, *Der moralische Diskurs über das medizinische Menschenexperimente im 19. Jahrhundert* (Stuttgart: Gustav Fischer, 1996), 231. Also Claudia Huerkamp, "Ärzte und Patienten: Zum strukturellen Wandel der Arzt-Patient-Beziehung vom ausgehenden 18. Bis zum frühen 20. Jahrhundert," in *Medizinische Deutungsmacht,* 57–73, especially 66. Also Lutz Sauerteig, "Ethische Richtlinien, Patientenrechte und ärztliches Verhalten bei der Arzneimittelerprobung," *Medizinhistorisches Journal* 35 (2000): 303–334; Sauerteig, *Krankheit, Sexualität, Gesellschaft,* 434–436.
16. Neill, "Transnationalism," 108.
17. Weindling, *Health, Race and German Politics,* 4.
18. Sauerteig, "'The Fatherland is in Danger,'" 76–92, 79, 77. Also Weindling, *Health, Race and German Politics,* 13, 90, 174, 177, 190; Vern Bullough and Bonnie Bullough, *Women and Prostitution: A Social History* (Buffalo, NY: Prometheus Books, 1987 [1978]), 232–233.
19. Neill, "Transnationalism," 108.
20. Claudia Huerkamp, "The Making of the Modern Medical Profession, 1800–1914: Prussian Doctors in the Nineteenth Century," in *German Professions, 1800–1950,* ed. Geoffrey Cooks and Konrad Jarausch (New York: Oxford University Press, 1990), 74.
21. Weindling, "Bourgeois Values, Doctors and the State," 198.
22. Huerkamp, *Der Aufstieg der Ärzte im 19. Jahrhundert. Vom gelehrten Stand zum professionellen Experten: Das Beispiel Preußens* (Göttingen: Vandenhoeck and Ruprecht, 1985), 68–70. See also Claudia Huerkamp, "Die preussisch-deutsche Ärzteschaft als Teil des Bildungsbürgertums," in *Bildungsbürgertum im 19. Jahrhundert,* vol. I, *Bildungssystem und Professionalisierung in internationalen Vergleich,* ed. Werner Conze and Jürgen Kocka (Stuttgart: Klett-Cotta, 1985), 358–387; Alfons Labisch, "Gesundheitskonzepte und Medizin im Prozeß der Zivilisation," in *Medizinische Deutungsmacht,* 15–36, especially 24; Alfons Labisch, "Doctors, Workers and the Scientific Cosmology of the Industrial World: The Social Construction of 'Health' and the 'Homo Hygienicus,'" *Journal of Contemporary History* 20 (1985): 599–615; Blackbourn, "The German Bourgeoisie," 11. See also Frevert, "Professional Medicine," 637–658.
23. Weindling, *Health, Race and German Politics,* 4.
24. Frevert, "Professional Medicine," 651; Abrams, "Prostitutes in Imperial Germany," 198.
25. Bleys, *The Geography of Perversion,* 152.
26. Blackbourn, "The German Bourgeoisie," 11.
27. Bleys, *The Geography of Perversion,* 152.
28. Weindling, "Bourgeois Values, Doctors and the State," 214; Peter Stachura, "Social Policy and Social Welfare in Germany from the Mid-nineteeth Century to the Present," in *Germany: A New Social and Economic History,* 230. For a brief history of the DGBG, see Lutz Sauerteig, "Die Deutsche Gesellschaft zur Bekämpfung der Geschlechtskrankheiten (DGBG), 1902–2002," *Aktuelle Dermatologie* 28 (2002): 393–397.
29. Huerkamp, *Der Aufstieg der Ärzte,* 172.

30. Weindling, "Bourgeois Values, Doctors and the State," 199; Göckenjan, "Wandlungen im Selbstbild des Arztes," 89–102; and Sauerteig, "Salvarsan und der 'ärztliche Polizeistaat,'" 193; Cornelia Regin, "Zwischen Angriff und Abwehr: Die Naturheilbewegung als medizinkritische Öffentlichkeit im Deutschen Kaiserreich," in *Medizinische Bewegung,* 40.
31. Sauerteig, *Krankheit, Sexualität, Gesellschaft,* 206, 293–297.
32. For example, see Dr. Wend, Bericht ueber den Gesundheitszustand der Matrosenartillerie-Abteilung Kiautschou 1. Januar–31. Maerz 1912, 1. April 1912, BArch-MA RM3/6764, 394–395. Also, Sauerteig, *Krankheit, Sexualität, Gesellschaft,* 344.
33. Sauerteig, *Krankheit, Sexualität, Gesellschaft,* 206, 293–297.
34. Ibid., 328–337, 295–297.
35. Schulte, *Sperrbezirke,* 32, 151–152; Abrams, "Prostitutes in Imperial Germany," 190; Sheldon Watts, *Epidemics and History. Disease, Power and Imperialism* (New Haven, CT: Yale University Press, 1997), 139–146; Mosse, *Nationalism and Sexuality,* 23–47; Bleys, *The Geography of Perversion,* 145, 189.
36. Martha Vicinus, "Sexuality and Power: A Review of Current Work in the History of Sexuality," *Feminist Studies* 8 (1982): 136. See also R. W. Connell, *Gender and Power: Society, the Person and Sexual Politics* (Stanford, CA: Stanford University Press, 1987), 137, 161, 168. Isabel Hull rightly notes in *Sexuality, State, and Civil Society* that this paradigm shift began in the late early modern period.
37. Mary Spongberg, *Feminizing Venereal Disease: The Body of the Prostitute in Nineteenth-Century Medical Discourse* (New York: New York University Press, 1997), 6, 35. See also Sander Gilman, *Difference and Pathology: Stereotypes of Sexuality, Race, and Madness* (Ithaca, NY: Cornell University Press, 1985), 94; Schulte, *Sperrbezirke,* 7; and Anita Ulrich, "Ärzte und Sexualität—am Beispiel der Prostitution," in *Medizinische Deutungsmacht,* 223–235, 229.
38. Sauerteig, "'The Fatherland is in Danger,'" 78–80. See also Lutz Sauerteig, "Medizin und Moral in der Syphilisbekämpfung," *Medizin, Gesellschaft und Geschichte* 19 (2000): 55–70; Jenders and Müller, *"Nur die Dummen sind eingeschrieben,"* 36; Bullough and Bullough, *Women and Prostitution,* 232–233; Hilpert-Fröhlich, *"Auf zum Kampfe wider die Unzucht,"* 19.
39. Spongberg, *Feminizing Venereal Disease,* 101, 6.
40. Evans, "Prostitution, State and Society," 110. See also Abrams, "Prostitutes in Imperial Germany," 191.
41. Abrams, "Prostitutes in Imperial Germany," 191. For a specific example, see the morals police regulations for Dortmund in Jenders and Müller *"Nur die Dummen sind eingreschrieben,"* 46–49.
42. Schulte, *Sperrbezirke,* 181–182.
43. Abrams, "Prostitutes in Imperial Germany," 194–197. See also Richard Evans, "Introduction: The 'Dangerous Classes' in Germany from the Middle Ages to the Twentieth Century," in *The German Underworld,* 13–14.
44. Abrams, "Prostitutes in Imperial Germany," 193. See also Evans, "Prostitution, State and Society," 112.
45. Sauerteig, *Krankheit, Sexualität, Gesellschaft,* 434; Sauerteig, "'The Fatherland is in Danger,'" 86–88.
46. Bullough and Bullough, *Women and Prostitution,* 232–233; Watts, *Epidemics and History,* 126, 158; Sauerteig, *Krankheit, Sexualität, Gesellschaft,* 32–33; and J. D. Oriel, *The Scars of Venus: A History of Venereology* (London: Springer-Verlag, 1994), 71–80, 131–134.
47. Weindling, "Bourgeois Values, Doctors and the State," 215.
48. "Feminist Perspectives on Objectification," *Stanford Encyclopedia of Philosophy,* 10 March 2010, revised 28 June 2011 (http://ww.plato.stanford.edu/entries/feminism-objectification/, accessed 19 September 2011).
49. Katja Sabisch, *Das Weib als Versuchsperson: Medizinische Menschenexperimente im 19. Jahrhundert am Beispiel der Syphilisforschung* (Bielfeld: Transcript, 2007), 12.

50. Barbara Elkeles, *Der moralische Diskurs,* 231; Jens Lachmund and Gunnar Stollberg, *Patientenwelten: Krankheit und Medizin vom späten 18. bis zum frühen 20. Jahrhundert im Spiegel von Autobiographien* (Opladen: Leske und Budrich, 1995), 18; Reinhard Spree, "Kurpfuscherei—Bekämpfung und ihre sozialen Funktion während des 19. und zu Beginn des 20. Jahrhunderts," in *Medizinische Deutungsmacht,* 113–114; and Sauerteig *Krankheit, Sexualität, Gesellschaft,* 82–83. Sauerteig, however, only suggests the idea of the objectification of patients, and hence underdevelops this phenomenon.
51. James Scott, *Seeing Like a State: How Certain Schemes to Improve the Human Condition Have Failed* (New Haven, CT: Yale University Press, 1998), 77, 81–82; David Kertzer and Dominique Arel, "Censuses, Identity Formation, and the Struggle for Political Power," in *Census and Identity: The Politics of Race, Ethnicity, and Language in National Censuses,* ed. David Kertzer and Dominique Arel (Cambridge: Cambridge University Press, 2002), 2, 6; and Talal Asad, "Ethnographic Representation, Statistics, and Modern Power," in *From the Margins: Historical Anthropology and Its Futures,* ed. Brian Axel (Durham, NC: Duke University Press, 2002), 82.
52. Axel Hüntelmann, *Hygiene im Namen des Staates: Das Reichsgesundheitsamt 1876–1933* (Göttingen: Wallstein, 2008), 213, 366–367. See also Hüntelmann, "Zwischen Kooperation und Kontrolle," in *Gesundheit und Staat: Studien zur Geschichte der Gesundheitsämter in Deutschland, 1870–1950,* ed. Axel Hüntelmann, Johannes Vossen, and Herwig Czech (Husum: Matthiesen, 2006), 26.

Chapter 2

Male Colonial Sexuality

The acquisition of overseas territories provided German men with increased opportunities to quench their desire not only for land, freedom, and adventure,[1] but also for sexual gratification. Edward Said pointed out that "the Orient was a place where one could look for sexual experience unobtainable in Europe."[2] Similarly, Ronald Hyam, writing about the British Empire, wrote that "empire unquestionably gave them an enlarged field of opportunity. Greater space and privacy were often available; inhibitions relaxed. European standards might be held irrelevant. Abstinence was represented as unhealthy in a hot climate. Boredom could constitute an irresistible imperative."[3] The circumstances in the German colonies were no different.[4]

As a matter of fact, contemporaries believed that the colonial environment heightened male sexuality. This was attributed to the climate and the example of the autochthonous populations. Some experts even argued that due to this situation, it was necessary for European men not to suppress their sexual drive. Otherwise, they would suffer serious consequences to their nervous systems or engage in undesirable debaucheries, such as homosexuality or masturbation.[5]

Others, however, did not agree with this assessment. In fact, some colonial officials and supporters believed that the colonial environment undermined the colonizers' ability to resist the attractiveness of indigenous women. This was merely another indication that tropical climates contributed to the overall degeneration of the white race. Increasingly, physicians published literature on the dangers "of intellectual and sexual degeneration caused by the physical and social climate of the tropics." This would ultimately undermine the supposed racial

Notes for this section begin on page 30.

purity of Europeans.[6] Regardless, though, of the perspective on European sexual liaisons with indigenous women, all agreed that the colonial setting significantly influenced male sexuality.

Most Europeans also concurred that non-European populations possessed an overactive sex drive.[7] The cultural historian Sander Gilman argued that "the view that the races were inherently different rested to no little extent on … sexual difference." For many Europeans, especially those in German-speaking countries, female black sexuality was embodied in the popular image of the "Hottentot Venus." In the first half of the nineteenth century, she became an object of desire among Europeans.[8] Even more beautiful than blacks were the Polynesians, in particular Samoans, at least according to contemporary accounts. Robert Tobin convincingly argues that the Germans developed a strong affinity for the Samoan people, who were often contrasted with the appearance of black indigenous populations, which further highlighted the "exceptional beauty" of the Samoans.[9] Nonetheless, regardless of their skin color, contemporary observers took great lengths to describe in detail the sexual practices of non-European peoples, such as polygamy and promiscuity,[10] in an effort to demonstrate their sexual rapacity.

In such a situation, white males often turned to indigenous women for sexual gratification. In fact, they were the primary option in lands were European women were conspicuously, but often consciously, absent. Due to climatic and financial concerns, most Europeans in Germany's overseas territories were male. Throughout Europe,[11] climate was often given as a reason why women should not go to the colonies, especially to those territories with a more tropical environment. Lajos Biró, a Hungarian naturalist and ethnographer, lived in German New Guinea for six years (1896–1902). He stated that "'owing to the extremely bad health-conditions the idea was then prevalent among men of European origin that a decent man must not take a European wife there because, given the disease-inducing climate that that area is subject to, this might even be considered an attempted murder.'"[12] A similar view was held by the governor of German Samoa, Wilhelm Solf (1900–1911). Though the climatic debates focused on both men and women, they tended to question primarily the fertility and constitution of women, but not those of men.[13]

Economics was another rationale given for limiting white female settlement in the colonies. According to the *German Colonial Encyclopedia,* "Because the maintenance of a European employee in the tropics is substantially more expensive than in Europe, the aim is ever more prominent both in private as well as in public enterprises to use only Europeans in managerial or oversight positions."[14] This was especially true for those regions that were acquired primarily for economic exploitation and not settlement purposes, such as Togo and New Guinea. In fact, the New Guinea Company only contracted unmarried men. Such a policy was not uncommon in other European colonies, such as the Dutch East Indies.

Thus, European men found themselves in an environment almost bereft of or with very limited numbers of white women. For example, even near the end of effective German control in 1913, there were 2,678 single men and only 374 single white women in German East Africa; in Togo 245 single men and 30 unmarried women; in Cameroon 1,286 single white men and only 58 single women; in German Southwest Africa 6,016 unmarried men and 900 single women; in New Guinea 826 single men to 161 unmarried white women; and in Samoa 221 unmarried men and 34 single women.[15] In Qingdao, there were 979 white men and 203 women in 1910.[16] Thus, the ratio of single white men to white women in East Africa was 7 to 1; in Togo 8 to 1; in Cameroon it was a staggering 22 to 1; in New Guinea 5 to 1; in Samoa 6.5 to 1, and in Qingdao almost 5 to 1. In the primary settlement colony of German Southwest Africa, the ratio was just under 7 to 1, even after the efforts of an organized program promoting female immigration to the colony. [17]

However, there was an abundance of indigenous women. Although no accurate statistics exist, the number of indigenous women far outnumbered the number of white males in the territories.[18] And, European men did find them attractive.[19] Moreover, as in other European colonies, numerous locations existed that offered opportunities for sexual contact between white men and indigenous women. For instance, plantations, trading posts, military compounds, mission posts, and settler communities provided locales for European men to have sex with autochthonous women.[20]

One of the more common ways European men gained access to autochthonous women was through rape, which also became a way for them to establish a new order in the colonial environment. R. W. Cornell noted that because "hegemonic masculinity in the metropole became more subject to rationalization" in the course of industrialization and modernization, "violence and license were" consequently "pushed to the colonies." The existing unbalanced sex ratio in the colonies allowed then for "a cultural masculinization of the frontier."[21] Violence, including rape, was one way for men to establish the "stability of colonial society," with themselves at the apex and indigenes below.[22]

Not surprisingly, the instances of rape in the colony were frequent.[23] One missionary in German New Guinea reported, "It was … fortunate that the natives in the beginning fearfully protected their wives and daughters from the evil traps of the whites,"[24] intimating that local leaders feared for the well-being of their women. In Southwest Africa, the historian Wolfram Hartmann suggested that local chiefs might have offered their women to passing Europeans in an attempt to prevent possible rape. He argued, though, that this was "for the women nothing other than male sanctioned rape."[25] Meanwhile in Togo, colonial administrators, including the governor, Herzog zu Mecklenburg (1912–1914), were "implicated in statutory rape and the officially prescribed procurement of African women and girls for intercourse."[26] On numerous occasions, indigenous minors throughout Germany's colonies were the objects of white male lust.[27]

The frequency of rape incidents increased as Germany more firmly established control over its colonies, and hence over the autochthonous populations. Peter Sebald argued that after the Germans conquered the coastal and interior parts of

Togo, African women were either forced or threatened with force to sleep with German men. He even contended that some were kept as an "African Harem at the military post,"[28] thus ensuring a ready supply of female sex partners. The forced recruitment of indigenous women for sex became so severe that Colonial Director Dr. Stübel issued a directive prohibiting such actions on the part of colonial authorities.[29]

Similar to other European colonies,[30] perhaps the most visible form of sexual contact between European men and indigenous women was concubinage.[31] A German settler in German East Africa stated that if a white man "was not married … he had a *bibi,* a black concubine."[32] In Cameroon, leading colonial administrators encouraged cohabitation between European men and indigenous women.[33] In the Pacific, the historian Hermann Hiery pointed out that "the practice of co-habitation between European men and indigenous women was certainly the rule."[34] Specifically in New Guinea, many traders and plantation owners had "laundresses," who were more likely to be "sexual partners and local advisors than laborers."[35] Some Europeans went beyond concubinage to actually enter into marriages with indigenous women.

In most cases, cohabitation and marriage were most likely a matter of convenience. For example, wives or mistresses would care for the man's household. As the Hungarian Biró in New Guinea explained, "Our wives were expected to do the chores, to keep our clothes in order, to see to it that the dirty linen were washed in time and clean dresses were always on hand."[36] Moreover, such relationships provided European men with ready access to female companionship—i.e., a way to satisfy their sexual desire. In addition, entering into such relationships had the potential to increase one's survival chances and prestige. By marrying or cohabiting with local women, European men gained access to indigenous knowledge and networks, which often played a significant survival tactic. For example, in German New Guinea, Pieter Hanson had nine wives, whom he either purchased or received for services rendered. These wives became a way for him to survive and be successful as a trader on the island of Witu. In Africa, such unions could also significantly improve the economic situation of white men. According to Friedrich von Lindequist, governor of German Southwest Africa (DSWA) (1905–1907), marriages to local women would give them access to local information and to land.[37]

Another means by which European men gained sexual access to indigenous women was through prostitution. This type of sexual contact was common throughout the European colonial setting,[38] primarily due to the common, though not shared, belief that males needed an outlet for their insatiable sex drive. When concubinage or marriage were not options or desired, prostitution was a practical alternative and, according to contemporary beliefs, was certainly preferable to same-sex relations and masturbation.[39]

Prostitution existed in the territories since the early days of German colonialism. However, it took on increased importance as German views of concubinage and miscegenation changed. This was especially true after some of the colonies, in particular those seen as more suitable for European settlement, such as Southwest Africa, East Africa, and Samoa, experienced increased immigration, above all of German women. Thus, as Germany increased its control over its possessions, the introduction of German values and norms followed. These norms, including bourgeois notions of respectability and marriage, blended with European concepts of race and degeneration. Consequently, concerns arose over male sexuality, in particular their choice of sexual partner and the outcomes of such relationships.[40]

The wrong choice—i.e., a non-European woman—threatened German racial purity and superiority in the colonies, and hence, German claims of domination. This was especially true because some staunch nationalists and colonial enthusiasts, including prominent German colonial officials, believed that German men in relationships with local women would go "native," i.e., sink to the level of the woman. "The woman … [does] not rise to the educational level of the man … , but rather the man sinks back to that of the woman. His house does not become a place of German ways and German family life, but rather he comes down in the world and degenerates more or less in his hut that maintains its mark through the essence of the woman and finally pulls the man down … to the level and sphere in which the woman was born and feels whole."[41] In other words, though perceived to be initially the dominant partner, white men in the German territories would ultimately become "conquered" by living with an indigenous woman—i.e., he would lose his European traits. Such thinking rested upon the belief that the domestic sphere belonged to the woman.[42] And these women, though not explicitly stated, could not conform to middle-class norms of the family because of their race.

The biggest cause for alarm, though, was the progeny from these relationships, especially because of German citizenship laws. According to German law, the children of German men automatically received their father's citizenship. Consequently, the "male half-castes would be eligible for conscription and be able to occupy public office,"[43] including even the governorship. If that was the case, the colonies would be lost to Germany because the next generation would be raised by their "native" mothers, and hence would not be true Germans.[44] Such a situation, according to contemporaries, undermined not only "the purity of the German race … but [also] the power of the white man."[45] They were the embodiment of "the moral and cultural degradation experienced by white men who lived with 'native' women," and hence "they represented all that was bad in German society."[46]

Many colonial officials and supporters agreed that it was imperative to address these challenges to German authority. However, the actual responses to miscegenation and the concomitant offspring varied. In those colonies with the relatively largest white populations, it was decided to separate the races. Therefore, in Southwest Africa (1905), East Africa (1906), and Samoa (1912), mixed marriages were banned, though many jurists considered this measure illegal. Moreover, in Southwest Africa, Germany's largest settler colony, those who married or even cohabited with indigenous women were even excluded from political participation and social life. In the other colonies, marriage and cohabitation was discouraged, but often with little effect. At the very least, colonial authorities throughout Germany's possessions passed ordinances to obviate the threats from offspring from sexual encounters across the racial divide by relegating these children to the status of "native."[47] By doing so, they could not receive German citizenship and the privileges that went with it.

Therefore, as concubinage and miscegenation became increasingly less of an option for European men, the only two officially state-sanctioned options left to men were either marrying German women or engaging a prostitute. For racial purists, there should only be sexual relations between European men and women. In fact, they believed that when presented with a choice, German men would choose their "racial equal." In support of this idea, the German Colonial Society (DKG) and its women's auxiliary, the Women's League of the German Colonial Socicty (FB), actively recruited and dispatched women to German Southwest Africa and eventually to Qingdao.[48] There were discussions about undertaking similar measures for Germany's other overseas territories that did not reach fruition. Although relatively well financed and supported, men still remained in the majority in DSWA as well as in the other colonies. Further, even when white women were available, many white men chose not to marry them.[49]

Thus, for many white men, the only real publicly permissible option was turning to a prostitute for their sexual gratification. Thus, while in some places laws and social constraints were implemented to segregate the races spatially, including at the level of permanent relationships, no policies were enacted to prevent sexual contact of a casual nature. Indeed, sex in the colonies was one area in which the races were not separated. In fact, it was a move advocated in many of the colonies.[50]

However, some German politicians criticized this state of affairs. Georg Ledebour, a Social Democratic representative in the German parliament (*Reichstag*), condemned the 1912 mixed-marriage ban in Samoa. He argued that because the sexual instinct could not be extinguished white men would be forced to seek sexual gratification through prostitution. "The Samoan women are degraded to some extent to a herd of prostitutes for the white government officials and white planters. That is a necessary consequence of such a barbaric decree."[51]

Such a situation was undoubtedly made possible by the racial and sexual inequality of the colonial situation, which included certain assumptions about indigenous sexuality. Although not ideal for racial purists, such sexual encounters at least did not approximate a formal relationship. Moreover, prostitutes could be marginalized through regulations like their counterparts in Germany and other European colonies were.[52] Essentially, then, white male sexuality was redirected. "In earlier years, the European more often sought a certain native women to engage; he had a black wife. Due to the influence of public opinion in Germany, … the European has broken himself of this habit. This has had the practical result that the white increasingly looks elsewhere for his sexual gratification, and consequently is directed to the black Venus vulgivaga."[53] Therefore, as in the metropole, prostitution constituted a "necessary evil,"[54] for it provided the least harmful outlet for male sexuality. In addition, it relieved men of taking any responsibility for their actions, especially if a child was produced.[55]

In the sexual hierarchy of the colonial environment, indigenous males occupied an ambiguous position. In terms of gender, they were seen as the dominant partner, but with respect to race, they were subordinate to whites. Such a perspective manifested itself through the pathologization of their sexuality and the limitations placed on their choice of sexual partners. Like non-European women, autochthonous males were largely viewed as sexualized. Not only were they seen as aggressively potent, they also were "irrational, impulsive and instinct driven."[56] In other words, they possessed a "'female' [sexual] volatility."[57] From the perspective of white men, this perspective necessitated a controlling and channeling of indigenous male sexuality. First and foremost, this entailed maintaining a racial and spatial barrier between autochthonous men and white women. At the same time, because these men would ostensibly need a non-European sexual partner, they required access to either a non-European wife or prostitute, or, as many German colonial doctors reported, both because they were often seen as synonymous.[58] Like with white men, such partners were certainly preferable to other men or even masturbation. Moreover, such a view justified and upheld white, heterosexual male rule in the European colonial setting.[59]

Notes

1. Johannes Does, *Ein alter Afrikaner* (Wismar: Hinstorffsche Verlagsbuchhandlung, 1913), 379–380; cited in John Noyes, "Wide Open Spaces and the Hunger for Land: Production of Space in the German Colonial Novel," *Faultline: Interdisciplinary Approaches to German Studies* 1 (1992): 106–107.
2. Edward Said, *Orientalism* (New York: Vintage Books, 1979), 190.
3. Ronald Hyam, *Empire and Sexuality: The British Experience* (Manchester: Manchester University Press, 1990), 88.
4. See, for example, the description of the Pacific environment in E. Freiherr von Spiegel, *Meere, Inseln, Menschen. Vom Seekadetten zum U-Boot-Kommandanten* (Berlin: August Scherl, 1934), 159.
5. Ludwig Külz, *Blätter und Briefe eines eines Arztes aus dem tropischen Deutschafrika* (Berlin: Wilhelm Süsserott, 1906), 68; Dr. K. Hintze, "Welchen Einfluss hat das Tropenklima auf Angehörige der weissen Rasse?" *Archiv für Schiffs- und Tropen-Hygiene* 20, no. 6 (1916): 155. See also Pascal Grosse, *Kolonialismus, Eugenik und bürgerliche Gesellschaft in Deutschland 1850–1918* (Frankfurt: Campus, 2000), 90; Thomas Schwarz, "Die Kultivierung des kolonialen Behehrens—ein deutscher Sonderweg?" in *Kolonialismus als Kultur. Literature, Medien, Wissenschaft in der deutschen Gründerzeit des Fremden,* ed. Alexander Honold and Oliver Simons (Tübingen: A. Francke, 2002), 91; and Liesbeth Hesselink, "Prostitution: A Necessary Evil, Particularly in the Colonies. Views on Prostitution in the Netherlands Indies," in *Indonesian Women*

in Focus. Past and Present Notions, ed. Elsbeth Locher-Scholten and Anke Niehof (Dardrecht, Holland: Foris Publications, 1987), 208.

6. Stepan, "Biological Degeneration," 102–103. See also Schwarz, "Die Kultiverierung des kolonialen Begehrens," 92.
7. Joanna de Groot makes the connection in her "'Sex' and 'Race': The Construction of Language and Image in the Nineteenth Century," in *Sexuality and Subordination: Interdisciplinary Studies of Gender in the Nineteenth Century,* ed. Susan Mendus and Jane Rendall (London: Routledge, 1989), 89–128.
8. Sander Gilman, "Black Sexuality and Modern Consciousness," in *Blacks and German Culture,* ed. Reinhold Grimm and Jost Hermand (Madison: University of Wisconsin Press, 1986), 39. See also Sander Gilman, "Black Bodies, White Bodies: Toward an Iconography of Female Sexuality in Late Nineteenth-Century Art, Medicine, and Literature," *Critical Inquiry* 12, no. 1 (1985): 213, 216.
9. Robert Tobin, "*Venus von Samoa.* Rasse und Sexualität im deutschen Südpazifik," in *Kolonialismus als Kultur: Literatur, Medien, Wissenschaft in der deutschen Gründerzeit des Fremden,* ed. Alexander Honold and Oliver Simons (Tubingen: A. Francke Verlag, 2002), 192–220, especially 207–209. See also Roland Samulski, "Die 'Sünde' im Auge des Betrachters—Rassenmischung und deutsche Rassenpolitik im Schutzgebiet Samoa 1900 bis 1914," in *Raschenmischehen,* 332–333.
10. For example, see the descriptions in Erdland's account of his travels in the South Seas. August Erdland, *Die Marshall-Insulaner. Leben und Sitte, Sinn und Religion eines Südsee-Volkes* (Munster: Aschendorffsche Verlagsbuchhandlung, 1914), 118, 124, 131ff., 197, 266. For a more detailed scholarly account, see Amadou Booker Sadj, *Das Bild des Negro-Afrikaners in der Deutschen Kolonialliteratur (1884–1945). Ein Beitrag zur literarischen Imagologie Schwarzafrikas* (Berlin: Dietrich Reimer Verlag, 1985), 144–149.
11. Pascal Grosse, "Turning Native? Anthropology, German Colonialism, and the Paradoxes of the 'Acclimatization Question,' 1885–1914," in *Worldly Provincialism: German Anthropology in the Age of Empire,* ed. H. Glenn Penny and Matti Bunzl (Ann Arbor: University of Michigan Press, 2003), 192–196; Ann Stoler, "Making Empire Respectable: The Politics of Race and Sexual Morality in 20th-Century Colonial Cultures," *American Ethnologist* 16 (November 1989): 650.
12. Lajos Biró, *My Papuan Wives,* cited in Gàbor Vargyas, *Data on the Pictorial History of North-East Papua New Guinea* (Budapest: Ethnographical Institute of the Hungarian Academy of Sciences, 1986), 41.
13. Evelyn Wareham, *Race and Realpolitik: The Politics of Colonisation in German Samoa* (Frankfurt: Peter Lang, 2002), 79. For a broader overview of the debates over climate, see, for example, Pascal Grosse, *Kolonialismus,* 53–95; Stepan, "Biological Degeneration," 97–120; Pascal Grosse, "Turning Native?" 179–197; and Richard Eves, "Unsettling Settler Colonialism: Debates Over Climate and Colonization in New Guinea, 1875–1914," *Ethnic and Racial Studies* 28, no. 2 (March 2005): 304–330.
14. Cited in Peter Sebald, *Togo 1884–1914. Eine Geschichte der deutschen "Musterkolonie" auf der Grundlage amtlicher Quellen* (Berlin: Akademie Verlag, 1988), 261.
15. Reichskolonialamt, ed., *Die deutschen Schutzgebiete in Afrika und der Südsee 1912/13: Amtliches Jahresbericht* (Berlin: Ernst Siegfried Mittler and Sohn, 1914), 10, 14, 18, 22, 28, 34. These figures do not include the number of married men whose wives were not with them in the colonies. In 1913, these numbers were Samoa: 10; New Guinea: 37; Southwest Africa: 347; Togo: 19; Cameroon: 102; East Africa: 157.
16. Dr. Uthemann and Dr. Fürth, "Tsingtau. Ein kolonialhygienischer Rückblick auf die Entwicklung des Deutschen Kiautschousbeibietes," *Beihefte zum ASTH* 15, no. 4 (1911): 37.
17. For information on this, see Lora Wildenthal, *German Women for Empire, 1884–1945* (Durham, NC: Duke University Press, 2001), 131–168, especially 156, 167; Daniel Walther, "Gender Construction and Settler Colonialism in German Southwest Africa, 1894–1914,"

The Historian 66, no. 1 (Spring 2004): 11; Daniel Walther, *Creating Germans Abroad: Cultural Policies and National Identity in Namibia* (Athens: Ohio University Press, 2002), 48–51; Krista O'Donnell, "The Colonial Woman Question: Gender, National Identity, and Empire in the German Colonial Society Female Emigration Program, 1896–1914," PhD dissertation (SUNY Binghamton, 1996).

18. Even by 1913, no real reliable statistics existed for the indigenous population in Germany's colonies. Even when figures were published, most colonial authorities knew they were not accurate and hence of no real use. Nonetheless, even though they are poor figures, they do demonstrate that the indigenous population far outnumbered the European one; thus, the assertion that there were more native women than single European men remains valid. For example, for Cameroon, it was estimated that the non-European population was 2.65 million in 1911. In German East Africa the population was roughly 4 million in 1913. In 1913, the indigenous population in Togo was estimated to be just over 1 million; in German New Guinea it was around 600,000. *Die deutschen Schutzgebiete in Afrika und der Südsee 1912/13,* 45, 58; Rudin, *Germans in the Cameroons,* 102; Juhani Koponen, *Development for Exploitation: German Colonial Policy in Mainland Tanzania, 1884–1914* (Helsinki: Tiedekirja, 1994), 588.
19. Daniel Walther, "Race, Sex, and Empire: White Male Sexuality and the 'Other' in Germany's Colonies," *German Studies Review* 33, no. 1 (February 2010): 51.
20. Hyam discusses similar locations for sexual interactions between Europeans and non-Europeans. Hyam, *Empire and Sexuality,* 91–114. For the specific case of German Southwest Africa, see Wolfram Hartmann, "Sexual Encounters and Their Implications on an Open and Closing Frontier: Central Namibia from the 1840s to 1905," PhD dissertation (Columbia University, 2002), 189–211.
21. R. W. Connell, *Masculinities* (Berkeley: University of California Press, 1995), 194.
22. David Kenosian, "The Colonial Body Politic: Desire and Violence in the Works of Gustav Frenssen and Hans Grimm," *Monatshefte* 89 (1997): 185–189. See also Andrea Smith, "Not an Indian Tradition: The Sexual Colonization of Native Peoples," *Hypatia* 18, no. 2 (2003): 76, 80.
23. For more on this, see Birthe Kundrus, *Moderne Imperialisten. Das Kaiserreich im Spiegel seiner Kolonien* (Cologne: Böhlau, 2003), 224, note 22; Bettina Zurstrassen, "Die Steuerung und Kontrolle der kolonialen Verwaltung und ihrer Beamten am Beispiel des 'Schutzgebietes' Togo (1884–1914)," PhD dissertation (Universität der Bundeswehr, 2005), 76–77; Walther, "Sex, Race, and Empire," 52–53. For an examination of same-sex rape in Germany's colonies, see Heike Schmidt, "Colonial Intimacy: The Rechenberg Scandal and Homosexuality in German East Africa," *Journal of the History of Sexuality* 17, no. 1 (January 2008): 25–59.
24. Albert Hoffmann, *Lebenserinnerungen eines Rheinischen Missionars,* vol. I: *Auf dem Missionsfeld in Neu-Guinea* (Wuppertal: Verlag der Rheinischen Missionsgesellschaft, 1948), 153.
25. Wolfram Hartmann, "Eine *situation érotique et coloniale* im 19. Jahrhundert: Männer und Frauen im südwestlichen Afrika," in *Die (koloniale) Begegnung. AfrikanerInnen in Deutschland 1880–1945. Deutsche in Afrika 1880–1918,* ed. Marianne Bechhaus-Gerst and Reinhard Klein-Arendt (Frankfurt: Peter Lang, 2003), 138.
26. Horst Gründer, *Christliche Mission und deutscher Imperialismus. Eine politische Geschichte ihrer Beziehungen während der deutschen Kolonialzeit (1884–1914) under besonderer Berücksichtigung Afrikas und Chinas* (Paderborn: Ferdinand Schöningh, 1982), 178; Schmidt, "Colonial Intimacy," 25, note 1. See also Zurstrassen, "Die Steuerung und Kontrolle," 76–77.
27. For example, Strafsache gegen Dimitris Sametes, Imperial Bezirksamt Windhuk, 27 November 1908, BArch R1001/4892, 16–17; Strafsache gegen Josef Scharbatke, Bezirksgericht Swakopmund, 18 September 1908, BArch R1001/4888, 4; Winterfeld to RKA, 8 April 1908, BArch R1001/4827, 3–4.
28. Peter Sebald, "Kolonialregime und Mischlinge. Das Beispiel der deutschen Kolonie Togo 1884–1914," in *Rassendiskriminierung, Kolonialpolitik und ethnisch-nationale Identität. Referate des 2. Internationalen Kolonialgeschichtlichen Symposiums 1991 in Berlin,* ed. Wilfried Wagner (Münster: Lit Verlag, 1992), 113.

29. Martha Mamozai, *Schwarze Frau, weiße Herrin. Frauenleben in den deutschen Kolonien* (Reinbek: Rowohlt, 1989), 128–129; Zurstrassen, "Die Steuerung und Kontrolle," 77, note 286; Matthias Erzberger, *Die Kolonial-Bilanz. Bilder aus der deutschen Kolonialpolitik auf Grund der Verhandlungen des Reichstags im Sessionsabschnitt 1905/06* (Berlin: Germania, 1906), 10.
30. For instance, see Stoler, "Making Empire Respectable," 637; and Alice Conklin, "Redefining 'Frenchness': Citizenship, Race Regeneration, and Imperial Motherhood in France and West Africa, 1914–40," in *Domesticating the Empire: Race, Gender, and Family Life in French and Dutch Colonialism,* ed. Julia Clancy-Smith and Frances Gouda (Charlottesville: University of Virginia Press, 1988), 76.
31. For more on this, see Walther, "Sex, Race, and Empire."
32. Burkhard Vieweg, *Macho Porini. Die Augen im Busch. Kauschukpflanzer Karl Vieweg in Deutsch-Ostafrika Authentische Berichte 1910–1919* (Weikersheim: Markgraf Verlag, 1996), 176.
33. Max Buchner, *Kamerun: Skizzen und Betrachtungen* (Leipzig: Duncker and Humbolt, 1887), 154–155; Rudin, *Germans in the Cameroons,* 304–305.
34. Hermann Hiery, "Germans, Pacific Islanders and Sexuality: German Impact and Indigenous Influence in Melanesia and Micronesia," in *European Impact and Pacific Influence: British and German Colonial Policy in the Pacific Islands and the Indigenous Response,* ed. Herman Hiery and John MacKenzie (London: Tauris Academic Studies, 1997), 302; Hermann Hiery, *Das Deutsche Reich in der Südsee (1900–1921). Eine Annäherung an die Erfahrungen verschiedener Kulturen* (Göttingen: Vandenhoeck & Ruprecht, 1995), 40–41.
35. Vargyas, *Data on the Pictorial History,* 43, 44. See also Hiery, *Das Deutsche Reich in der Südsee,* 54.
36. Vargyas, *Data on the Pictorial History,* 46.
37. Paul Kohlstock, *Ratgeber für die Tropen. Handbuch für Ausrüstung, Aufenthalt, Reisen und Behandlung von Krankheiten,* 3rd ed. (Stettin: Hermann Peters Verlag, 1910), 118; Hiery, *Das Deutsche Reich in der Südsee,* 48, 45; Burkhard Vieweg, *Big Fellow Man. Muschelgeld und Südseegeister. Authentische Berichte aus Deutsch-Neuguinea 1906–1909* (Weikersheim: Margraf, 1990), 272–273; Hiery, "Germans, Pacific Islanders and Sexuality," 301; Sebald, "Kolonialregime und Mischlinge," 110; Hartmann, "Eine *situation érotique et coloniale,*" 137, 140–141; Lindequist, Vertrauliche Rundverfügung an die Bezirksämter, 20 December 1905, BArch R8023/175. See also Richard Pierard, "The Transportation of White Women to German Southwest Africa, 1898–1914," *Race* (1970–1971): 317; Wildenthal, *German Women,* 109.
38. For the case of the British Empire, which is the more thoroughly researched, see Hyam, *Empire and Sexuality*; and Levine, *Prostitution, Race, and Politics.*
39. Hesselink, "Prostitution: A Necessary Evil," 206–207, 208–209. See also Philippa Levine, "'A Multitude of Unchaste Women': Prostitution in the British Empire," *Journal of Women's History* 15, no. 4 (Winter 2004): 160; Walther, "Sex, Race, and Empire," 58; Hannecke Ming, "Barracks-Concubinage in the Indies, 1887–1920," *Indonesia* 35 (1983): 63–93, 70; Ann Stoler, *Race and the Education of Desire: Foucault's History of Sexuality and the Colonial Order of Things* (Durham, NC: Duke University Press, 1997), 129.
40. See Walther, *Creating Germans Abroad,* 46–63; and Kundrus, "'Weiß und herrlich,'" 44. Both discuss male sexuality within the context of gender and not specifically through the lens of sexuality. For a discussion of respectability and colonialism, see Woodruff Smith, "Colonialism and the Culture of Respectability," in *Germany's Colonial Pasts,* ed. Eric Ames, Marcia Klotz, and Lora Wildenthal (Lincoln: University of Nebraska Press, 2005), 3–20.
41. Quoted in Theodor Leutwein, *Elf Jahre Gouverneur in Deutsch-Südwestafrika* (Berlin: Mittler and Sohn, 1906), 232–233.
42. See, for example, Karin Hausen, "Family and Role-Division: The Polarisation of Sexual Stereotypes in the Nineteenth Century—An Aspect of the Dissociation of Work and Family Life," in *The German Family: Essays on the Social History of the Family in Nineteenth- and Twentieth-Century Germany,* ed. Richard Evans and W. R. Lees (London: Groom Helm, 1981), 51–83.
43. Oskar Hintrager to AA, 5 October 1905, BArch N1037/8; Tecklenburg to AA, 23 October 1905, BArch R1001/5417.

44. Lora Wildenthal, "Race, Gender, and Citizenship in the German Colonial Empire," in *Tensions of Empire: Colonial Cultures in a Bourgeois World,* ed. Frederick Cooper and Ann Stoler (Berkeley: University of California Press, 1997), 264; Walther, *Creating Germans Abroad,* 35.
45. Hintrager to AA, 5 October 1905; Tecklenburg to AA, 23 October 1905.
46. Walther, *Creating Germans Abroad,* 35.
47. Wildenthal, "Race, Gender, and Citizenship," 267. See also Harald Sippel, "'Im Interesse des Deutschtums und der weißen Rasse': Behandlung und Rechtswirkungen von 'Mischehen' in den Kolonien Deutsch-Ostafrika und Deutsch-Südwestafrika," *Jahrbuch für afrikanisches Recht* 9 (1995): 123–157; Sippel, "Rechtspolitische Ansätze zur Vermeidung einer Mischlingsbevölkerung in Deutsch-Südwestafrika," in *Raschenmischehen,* 138–164; and Wareham, *Race and Realpolitik,* 138–143; Walther, *Creating Germans Abroad,* 40, 41, 42; Sebald, "Kolonialregime und Mischlinge," 113–114, 115.
48. Wildenthal, *German Women,* 131–168, especially 156, 167; Walther, "Gender Construction," 11; Walther, *Creating Germans Abroad,* 46–53; O'Donnell, "The Colonial Woman Question"; Pierard, "The Transportation of White Women," 317–322; DKG, Tsingtao Chapter to DKG, Berlin, 20 October 1903, BArch R8023/186, 2–3; DKG to Hamburg-Amerika-Linie, 18 August 1905, BArch R8023/186, 74; DKG to Engels, Chair Tsingtao Chapter, 25 February 1908, BArch R8023/186, 38.
49. For statistics regarding German Southwest Africa, see Walther, *Creating Germans Abroad,* 58; O'Donnell, "The Colonial Woman Question," 244.
50. Peter Sebald, "Kolonialregime und Mischlinge," 115; Claudia Essner, "'Wo Rauch ist, da ist auch Feuer': Zu den Ansätzen eines Rassenrechts für die Deutschen Kolonien," in *Rassendiskriminierung, Kolonialpolitik und ethnisch-nationale Identität. Referate des 2. Internationalen Kolonialgeschichtlichen Symposiums 1991 in Berlin,* ed. Wilfried Wagner (Hamburg: Lit, 1992), 154, 156, 157.
51. *Verhandlungen des Reichtags,* 1912, vol. 238, 98 (http://www.reichstagsprotokolle.de/Blatt_k13_bsb00003350_00106.html). Wolfgang Eckart notes a similar situation in China: *Medizin und Kolonialismus,* 479.
52. Sauerteig, *Krankheit, Sexualität, Gesellschaft,* 59; Stoler, *Race and the Education of Desire,* 129, 179; Ming, "Barracks-Concubinage," 83; Hesselink, "Prostitution: A Necessary Evil," 208.
53. *MB 1907/08* (1909): 200–201.
54. I borrow this term from Hesselink, "Prostitution: A Necessary Evil," who uses it to describe a similar situation in the Dutch Indies.
55. Walther, *Creating Germans Abroad,* 41; Essner, "'Wo Rauch ist,'" 154.
56. El-Tayeb, "Verbotene Begegnungen," 90.
57. Bleys, *Geography of Perversion,* 172. For a general discussion of this, see Frantz Fanon, *Black Skin, White Masks* (New York: Grove Press, 1982).
58. El-Tayeb, "Verbotene Begegnungen," 85–95; Adjaï Paulin Oloukpona-Yinnon, "Zur Begegnung zwischen Weiß und Schwarz in Deutschland im kolonialen Kontext. Das Beispiel von Togoern im kaiserlichen Deutschland," in *Die (koloniale) Begegnung,* 238–240; Verena Westermann, "Eine fast vergessene Einwanderung. AfrikanerInnen in Hamburg 1884–1945," in *Branntwein, Bibeln und Bananen. Der Deutsche Kolonialismus in Afrika—eine Spurrensuche,* ed. Heiko Möhle (Hamburg: Verlag Libertäre Assoziation, 1999), 87–88; and Lora Wildenthal, *German Women,* 111–117. See also Kundrus, *Moderne Imperialisten,* 224, note 23; *MB 1905/06* (1907): 198; *MB 1908/09* (1910): 511; *AkG* (1898): 634.
59. Fatima El-Tayeb similarly asserts that German males used the protection of white women as a justification for white male rule and the subjugation of indigenous men, but her interpretation ignores the gendered role of indigenous men in autochthonous societies as perceived by Europeans. El-Tayeb, "Verbotene Begegnungen," 85–95. For other European colonies, see Stoler, *Race and the Education of Desire.*

Chapter 3

PROSTITUTION IN GERMANY'S COLONIES

As several scholars have already demonstrated, the introduction of European rule and the concomitant changes to the local economies opened up new possibilities for indigenous women to earn an income. Indeed, the disruption of preexisting economies, the proletarianization of indigenous societies, and the introduction of migrant labor either provided women with opportunities to attain financial independence or required them to support their families or themselves. One of the easiest ways to earn money was through prostitution, especially due to the presence of a disproportionately large number of single men.[1] And, either on their own volition or forced by family members, or through the international trade of white and Asian women, there was more than a sufficient supply of prostitutes in all of Germany's colonies serving either or both white or non-Western clients.

The earlier reports from the African colonies first placed prostitution primarily in coastal cities. For instance, in the 1890s colonial officials reported the presence of prostitutes in the German East African ports of Dar es Salaam (the colonial capital) and Tanga[2]; Lomé (the colonial capital beginning in 1897) in Togo[3]; and Douala[4] (the primary port of entry for the territory) and Victoria (present-day Limbi, near the coast) in Cameroon. These harbor towns were the first places where Germany established itself in the colonies and were filled with large male populations, many of whom were there for short periods of time, in search of sexual gratification. Over time, these ports grew in size and significance, which further increased the population and sexual demand. For instance, the population of Dar es Salaam in East Africa was approximately 10,000 in 1894 (ca. 9,000 Africans, 400 Europeans, and 620 Indians). By 1913, the number of inhabitants had more than doubled to about 22,500 (ca. 19,000 Africans, 967 Europeans,

Notes for this section begin on page 46.

2,629 Indians, and 400 Arabs). The constructions of the central rail line contributed significantly to the growth of the city, bringing Africans from the interior and foreigners from abroad. Similarly, Douala, Cameroon, grew significantly. In the years after the establishment of the colony, it became the largest urban center in Cameroon, despite the Germans moving the administrative capital to Buea in 1901.[5]

Prostitution was also widespread in Southwest Africa, Germany's largest settlement colony. Already in 1893, the colony's first government physician noted that prostitution was practiced by both indigenous and white women in Groß-Windhoek (the territorial capital) and Klein-Windhoek. By the end of the decade, the chief medical officer for the colonial troops (*Schutztruppe*), Dr. Lübbert, noted that prostitutes not only worked in Windhoek (the colonial capital), but also Swakopmund (an important port of entry for the territory), Okahandja (just north of Windhoek in central Namibia), Omaruru (northwest of Okahandja), and Otjimbingwe (west and north of Windhoek) among other places,[6] a trend mirroring the expansion of German control in the region.

Indeed, as German control moved farther into the interior and efforts were made to integrate the local economies into the international economy, prostitution became more widespread. This not only resulted in more Europeans going to the colonies, but also in the integration of more indigenes into the colonial system. In East Africa, the medical reports often indicated that prostitution was present in the various military stations or German settlements throughout the colony. By 1912, a government report stated that prostitutes worked in twelve of the sixteen largest settlements in the colony. This included not only other coastal towns, such as Kilwa, Lindi, and Pangani, but also Iringa in the central part, Mwanza in the north on Lake Victoria, and as far west as Wilhelmsthal and Bismarckburg.[7]

Similarly, in German West African colonies of Togo and Cameroon, known prostitution gradually spread inland as German control extended itself. In Togo by the end of German colonial rule, public health officials reported the existence of prostitution in places such as Atakpame (north of Lomé) and Kamina, in central Togo. Already by 1909/10, reports in Cameroon revealed that prostitution had spread to the central part of the colony (to Lomie), the southwest (to Ebolowa), the northwest (to Dschang), the northeast (to Garua), the far northeast (to Kusseri, on lake Chad), and north central Cameroon (to Banyo).[8]

Often large influxes or concentrations of men resulted in an increase in prostitution. This was certainly the case during the Herero and Nama Wars (1904–1907) in DSWA. During that time, the rise in the number of prostitutes, especially those of European descent, increased significantly with the arrival of approximately 17,000 soldiers to fight the Herero and Nama.[9] These men were either single or unaccompanied by spouses or girlfriends. The appearance of prostitution also accompanied large construction sites, such as the building of railroads. In Togo, for example, "as the number of men in Lomé had grown to more than 100 men with the construction of transportation facilities, the government opened in 1909 a bordello for them ... with about 40 African prostitutes."[10] The railway doctor Krauss noted a similar situation in East Africa.[11]

There were basically two types of prostitution in Africa. The first form was more structured, meaning that there were specific, known locations where men could find prostitutes, where "women could be visited ... informally and formally."[12] These were the professional (*Berufs-* or *erwerbsmässige*) prostitutes. The other type was situational prostitution (*Gelegenheitsprostitution*).

In many of the larger settlements of German East Africa, professional prostitutes operated. For example, in 1911/12 Dar es Salaam, there were ten non-African prostitutes and thirty-one African prostitutes. The latter were first quartered (*kaserniert*) in specific indigenous houses belonging to the community. Eventually, these were replaced with a single elongated corrugated iron construction. There were also professional prostitutes working in Tanga, Iringa, and the distant settlements of Wilhelmsthal and Bismarckburg.[13]

Professional prostitutes also operated in West Africa. In Togo, for instance, they worked in such places as in Lomé, Anecho, and Atakpame. Colonial officials required those African prostitutes who were only available to white men to live and work in specific locations (*Kasernierung*) in these towns. In Lomé, these women were housed in a bordello, which was opened in 1909 to accommodate the increase in the number of white men working on the traffic facilities. In the beginning, forty African women worked there. Meanwhile in Cameroon, officials reported professional prostitutes working at least in Banyo in the north. Staff physician Dr. Jäger reported that in Kusseri many of the prostitutes were women connected to long-distance trade, which in that area meant that most of the men were traveling. In addition, military officials also noted that soldiers often engaged in presumably prostitutive sex with indigenous women while on patrol. The reports did not clarify whether these women were professional or opportunity prostitutes. By 1909, bordellos either existed in the colony or the Government Council in Buea (the capital) was considering introducing them.[14]

From the beginning of German settlement in Southwest Africa, indigenous settlements (*Werften*) were popular places to visit for commercial sex. These *Werften* "usually took the form of a grouping of shacks and hovels around the largest employers such as government, police, military, breweries and larger hotels. The earliest official manifestation of such prostitution" was recorded in 1893 Windhoek.[15] In 1901/02, one medical official reported that between seventy and eighty women's rooms (*Frauenzimmer*)—i.e., where prostitutes worked—existed in the capital. Their services were significantly less expensive than those provided by white prostitutes. According to Dr. Gustav Heim, an African prostitute in Windhoek charged only 20 Pfennings, while a white one demanded at least 20 Marks. No doubt that this had contributed to the state of affairs in 1905, when colonial police had to prohibit whites from entering indigenous locations during the night because the situation had gotten out of control.[16] Wolfram Hartmann characterized these locations as "huge whorehouse[s], [that were] ransacked nocturnally by drunken men, soldiers and settlers alike, in pursuit of sexual relief."[17]

As the white population grew, especially with the increase in the number of soldiers sent to the colony to fight the Nama and Herero during 1904–1907, so did the number of *Werften* they could visit. In some locations, such as in Okahandja, the African prostitutes occupied a specific location within the *Werft.*[18] However, in other places, in Windhoek for instance, this was not the case. According to Governor Theodor Seitz, "The accommodation of colored female prostitutes in special *Werften* or houses is simply impossible, it would lead to situations that would be worse than the existing ones."[19]

Around 1904, after the start of the Herero and Nama Wars, women of European descent worked more commonly as prostitutes in the colony. For example, in late 1904 Swakopmund, the local police sergeant, Weber, noted that three European prostitutes lived in a house owned by one innkeeper, two others by another innkeeper, and four in a house owned by a carpenter. Two additional prostitutes had gone on to Okahandja. That same year, "a larger number of prostitutes arrived here, of which six stayed in Swakopmund and the remaining traveled to Okahandja." Additional prostitutes were expected with the next steamer from Cape Town.[20]

Bordello-like establishments also existed in the colony, in places like Windhoek and Swakopmund, though not until after the beginning of the twentieth century. Indeed, as late as 1898/99, Dr. Lübbert regretted "that the introduction of bordellos according to foreign [i.e., German] standards" was not yet possible.[21] When they were finally permitted, the colonial government took "a certain *laissez-faire* approach" to such places.[22] The Austrian journalist Franz Seiner reported in late December 1902 the existence of a bordello located in a Windhoek hotel where he happened to be staying. He moved to a different one the next day.[23] From his description, though, it was not entirely clear whether or not the bordello was staffed by African or white women.

It appeared that it was not until after the beginning of wars in 1904 that professionally run European-type brothels operated and staffed by whites came into existence in Windhoek and Swakopmund. This was in no small part a response to the sudden influx of thousands of soldiers and sailors sent to the colony to fight.[24] Dr. Gustav Heim spoke of "a large, fine, under medical supervision bordello with about 4 prostitutes" in Windhoek.[25] It was unclear whether this was one of the two bordellos that operated in the northern part of the capital by two non-German, white women.[26] In Swakopmund, it appeared that "snazzy French women" had also set up business "under a corrugated iron shack" in order "to take the savings from upright Germans who came from the field," according to one contemporary. In addition, two French women had apparently run another bordello out of house.[27] By 1906, records indicated that at least one more bordello existed in Swakopmund, which was ostensibly owned by a German woman, Elsa Schmidt.[28] There was a desire to establish a bordello in the mining town of Tsumeb for whites only, but it ultimately failed because it was believed that its existence would contribute to a decline in sexual contact between whites and Africans. According to the local official, there were "enough opportunities for sexual intercourse for white workers in the bush."[29]

In order to avoid the harassment of respectable members of the white community, colonial authorities strictly regulated prostitutes' lives along lines similar to those that existed in Germany. Accordingly, officials issued guidelines on "where they could live and work as well as how they could dress and behave in public."[30] For instance, they could not live in bars or public entertainment localities. In fact, prostitutes needed police approval for their place of residence. Further, if more than one prostitute lived in the same house, each had to have her own room with no connecting doors or passages to the others. When in public, they had to dress appropriately and "the addressing of men on the street, the noticeable back and forth strutting, remaining on sidewalks as well as all other public behavior meant to attract men [was] forbidden." Finally, prostitutes in Swakopmund were required to submit to a weekly medical examination and to follow the physician's orders. Doctors were required to report their findings to the police.[31]

Officials also applied strict regulations to bordellos, where white prostitutes by at least 1909 were required to live and work. These ordinances stipulated that bordellos must lie outside the city and that the property must be separated from the street "with a massive, solid and about two meter high wall topped with either barbed wire or glass shards." In addition, the property was permitted only one entrance, and it had to be facing the street. After darkness, it was "to be illuminated with a visible … red lantern." Finally, the women's rooms had to be separated by solid walls.[32]

Those women who did not follow these regulations were subject to legal prosecution and imprisonment for up to six months. Foreign prostitutes—i.e., not German—could even be expelled from the territory if they caused a "public nuisance" or endangered "good morals."[33] In one case, three women wrote the Bezirks office that they had given up prostitution and had begun living and working in a bar. However, the local official warned them that they would still be under police supervision and would remain so until he had decided otherwise. They essentially ignored this and were indicted for not following the ordinances governing women under moral control (*Sittenkontrolle*), regulations that required them to have weekly medical exams and forbade them from living in a bar. In convicting the women, the judge based his decision on the fact "that a prostitute under moral control simply declaring she wants to give up prostitution is insufficient to release her from her … obligations. A declaration of the police that the control is canceled must supervene, otherwise every possibility of the supervision of prostitution would be fully illusionary."[34]

In 1910, the Territorial Council in DSWA discussed various options for controlling the spread of disease and limiting continued sexual relations between whites and Africans. One solution, forwarded by the farmer Schlettwein, was to require all African women to work in state run bordellos. He asserted that white males would not curb their sexual activities. He added that white women should not be used because it could undermine their position among Africans. This was a part of the ostensible attempt to turn African women into prostitutes. The only apparent outcome was increased state supervision of white prostitutes working in bordellos.[35]

During the Nama and Herero Wars, the concentration of African women in camps provided a source of sexual release for whites and a source of income for the indigenous women and sometimes their husbands. Many of these women, however, were most likely raped. Such sexual exchanges occurred primarily around Windhoek and Swakopmund, where large prisoner-of-war camps were built. In Windhoek, after soldiers had apparently begun on a large scale to force sexual services from women in various places, military officials established a so-called *Bordell-Werft* (bordello pontook) in an effort to gain more control over the situation. It was unclear whether the Ovaherero women working there provided their services willingly or not. The bordello only lasted for a short period of time.[36]

The second type of commercial sex practiced in the colonies was opportunity prostitution. It was in all probability the most prominent, but it was difficult to quantify exactly how widespread it was because these prostitutes did not register themselves. "Those who chose prostitution as an actual means of making money were outnumbered by those who were driven to it by poverty, as a means of survival."[37] Nonetheless, with the increase in predominantly white male settlement in the colonies, there were more opportunities for sexual contact. In DSWA, for instance, African women were drawn by employment opportunities to work for Europeans as housekeepers, "bar maids and in other occupations."[38] These work locations also became places for situational prostitution; their employers, white men, often visited them in the night or asked them to stay over. Prostitutive forms of sexual exchange also took place outside the larger settlement areas.[39] The journalist Seiner related such an incident on his travels through Southwest Africa. "As soon as it became dark, an older and four young Herero came and offered us a 'omakeintu' (woman, girl). The price 5 marks. Soon thereafter a young Herero appeared with his sister, a 17-year-old voluptuously developed girl, offered her to us, and demanded for the service half a plug of tobacco."[40]

Medical officials also reported the practice of opportunity prostitution in Germany's other African colonies. In East Africa reports stated that only situational prostitution existed in places such as Lindi and Moschi. Out of Togo came accounts of women engaged in situational prostitution, including in Lomé. In Douala, at least in the early 1900s, there were situational prostitutes,[41] while in Victoria a physician noted that this form of prostitution, which was described as "secret prostitution" (*Geheimprostitution*), was "widespread" there in 1905/06.[42]

Prostitution was also present in Germany's Pacific possessions. In Samoa, for instance, both professional and situational prostitution existed. However, according to government physician Dr. Schwesinger, there were only a few registered prostitutes, while the majority engaged in "secret prostitution," or opportunity prostitution.[43] In New Guinea, on the large European plantations in the Old Protectorate (which included Kaiser-Wilhelmsland, the Bismarck Archipelago, and the northern Solomon Islands—i.e., in Melanesia) prostitution was prevalent as a result of the large concentration of men, similar to the situation on other large plantations throughout the Pacific. Prostitution also existed in Germany's so-called Island Territories in Micronesia (such as the Caroline, Palau, Marshall, and Mariana Islands). For example, Dr. Born reported in 1902 that prostitution existed on the island of Yap in the West Carolines, but due to the minimal shipping traffic it would be easy to supervise.[44] By 1911/12, a colleague stated that prostitution, "in a European sense," did not exist anywhere else in the colony except in Rabaul.[45]

There, the colonial government had allowed the establishment of the colony's only bordello system. The first brothel in the territory was set up on the island of Matupit (at the mouth of Bismarck Bay and south of Rabaul) in the early 1900s. Realizing that suppressing prostitution was impossible due to the increasing number of whites who came to the island aboard ships and the large numbers of Chinese who lived there, Governor Albert Hahl (1902–1914) granted Ah Tam, a Chinese shipwright and merchant, the right to set up the bordello. He originally employed three Japanese prostitutes so as to avoid the use of indigenous women in the trade. In addition, such an agreement allowed the government to regulate the terms of their entry into the colony and their place of residence, which included regular medical examinations.[46]

In 1910, when the new capital was set up in Rabaul, Ah Tam moved his brothel there as well. According to medical records for 1911/12, eight to ten Japanese prostitutes worked there in two bordellos. By late 1913, the number of prostitutes had nearly tripled, with twenty to thirty prostitutes serving white and Chinese clients. However, by early 1914, apparently only seventeen prostitutes worked in the two brothels.[47]

In the German Kiautschou Bay concession in the northeastern province of Shandong, China, "wild prostitution" prospered.[48] This was a result of the presence of the well-paid "male, primarily unmarried [Chinese] worker population"[49] and the large number of unmarried sailors in the German garrison. In 1904, there were 574 European (not including the German sailors) and 25,521 Chinese men compared to only 195 European and 1,694 Chinese women. Considering the prevailing views of male sexuality, it was assumed these men would need a sexual outlet, and according to the documents, men did indeed seek prostitutes either in Qingdao, the administrative capital, or in villages surrounding it.[50]

In response to the increasing concerns over the spread of venereal diseases and assaults on European women, bordellos were established in the colony. For the Europeans, five official bordellos operated: two run by Japanese, two by Chinese, and one by a German. The number of Chinese brothels was not reported. Around 1900, most of the prostitutes were either Chinese, or Japanese, or Russian. However, a sharp division existed between the brothels that Europeans could visit and the ones Chinese could enter.[51] "The use of those houses frequented by indigenes by Europeans was totally banned. Those bordellos accessible only to the latter [i.e., Europeans] … were not allowed to receive visits from Chinese under the threat of severe penalties."[52] At times, though, because of lower costs, soldiers would visit less expensive houses not officially sanctioned by the government or even the "wild prostitutes" in the surrounding forests.[53] In a real sense, official actions contributed to the growing significance of a sexual milieu on the fringes of the safe sexual zone military authorities attempted to create. Thus, according to the sinologist Klaus Mühlhahn, "in a socially gray area sexual contacts were frequently sought."[54] Moreover, they could not be entirely controlled.

Nevertheless, as the situation in Qingdao revealed, there was a conscious attempt in some territories to separate the prostitutes visited by whites from those used by indigenes or non-Europeans. For instance, in Rabaul, the two brothels with Japanese prostitutes were only to admit nonindigenous males. In Lomé, Togo, a bordello for whites only was staffed by African prostitutes. Meanwhile, in Dar es Salaam and in several locations in Southwest Africa, white prostitutes serviced only white males. Indeed, when white prostitutes were involved, non-Europeans were strictly prohibited from using their services.

There were basically two reasons for this. The primary one was directly related to issues of health. The separation of facilities prevented non-Europeans, or at least indigenes, from transmitting VD to whites. This underscored the belief that indigenous populations were dirty and diseased. This perception, though, was not consistent across Germany's colonial empire. For example, in Qingdao, whites and Chinese visited separate bordellos, but in Rabaul they apparently went to the same ones. Also related to health was the condition that prostitutes in all bordellos that serviced whites had to undergo a regular examination, often on a weekly basis. In Qingdao, the brothels frequented by Chinese were not regulated in this manner. Thus, by housing these prostitutes in bordellos, colonial authorities could regulate those who provided the services, but also who solicited the services of whites or the equivalent of whites in order to maintain the health of the ruling population. However, near the end of German rule in New Guinea, indigenous men started visiting those brothels in Rabaul that were supposed to deny them entry.[55]

Another reason to segregate the locations where whites and nonwhites sought sexual gratification was to uphold the racial hierarchy. While not important to everyone, it was a concern for some, especially in Germany's largest settler colony, Southwest Africa. In his application to run a brothel in Seeheim near Keetmanshoop, Karl Bambers argued that "the establishment of a bordello [was] definitely necessary" not only "in the interest of public health" but also for "the preservation of the appearance of the whites." He noted that, according to doctors, numerous "native" women suffered from venereal diseases. Further, he argued that "the sexual intercourse of whites with natives does not contribute to raising the appearance of the white race with the latter."[56]

Even in the Pacific, a certain racial hierarchy was maintained. For instance, the colonial government in New Guinea in the 1906/07 annual report classified the Japanese as "persons of equal status" with Europeans, while it gave the Chinese the ambiguous category of "non-indigenous colored."[57] In Qingdao, the situation was more complex in that relations between Europeans and Chinese were not just founded on racial categories, but also included cultural and social factors. In addition, as part of the larger concern of preventing relationships between white women and non-Europeans, colonial authorities required white prostitutes to work in brothels so that they could prevent indigenes from soliciting the women. In Togo, in order to prevent the occurrence of such a situation, the colonial administration only permitted black prostitutes to work.[58] Due to demographics, there were not enough nonindigenous women to service all European men, just like there were not enough white women to serve as wives for white men.

As the European population grew and more and more indigenes became integrated into the global economy, there were both more white and non-Western men with disposable income and more women (both white and non-Western) willing to take it from them. The economic opportunities for women were often limited, and prostitution was usually more profitable than earning a wage.[59] As in other European colonies,[60] the reasons women engaged in prostitution varied, but could be reduced to three primary ones: they desired to earn an income for themselves or their families; family members forced them into it as a means of increasing family income; or the international trade in white and Asian women brought them into the profession. The first two were more common in Africa, at least among indigenous women, while the third pertained primarily to European and Asian women throughout Germany's possessions.

According to the historian Luise White, women in East Africa engaged in prostitution for one of three reasons: out of necessity (survival), to support fathers, and to gain independence. These "women [thus] saw prostitution as a reliable means of capital accumulation, not as a despicable fate or a temporary strategy." White noted that at times these different types overlapped and even merged into one another, though rarely in the case of women working for their families.[61] Other scholars noted similar reasons in other areas of Africa.[62]

In German Africa, there were several examples of women turning to prostitution in order to earn an income for themselves. As on observer noted in Southwest Africa, indigenous women preferred that "their men or relatives did not know of their side employment (*Nebenerwerb*) so that they did not have to share the earnings with them."[63] Missionaries in DSWA also noted that imprisoned Herero during the years of war in the early twentieth century apparently preferred to earn money by prostituting themselves to white men rather than having a husband.[64]

The money they earned could enable these women either to support themselves or their families. In some parts of Africa, the money made from prostitution was used to acquire land or livestock. This was often necessary as a result of European colonial policies that disadvantaged indigenous owners of land and livestock.[65] The German reports, however, disparaged the indigenous populations. For instance, in Cameroon one physician wrote that among the Ngumbas and Bulus around Grossbatanga, "the women [were] rented or lent out so that the husband [could] satisfy his need for rum."[66] In Southwest Africa, one settler insisted that many African families nourished themselves through prostitution. "Many men prefer not to work," Bambers, the man who wanted to open a bordello with white women, contended, "but rather to lead a comfortable life from the money which their wives and daughters earn through their filthy business."[67]

Admittedly, as the German sources indicated, some women in the African colonies engaged only in opportunity prostitution. White noted a similar experience in British East Africa. The two main reasons tended to be either to supplement one's income in a financial emergency or to get one through a period of poverty. Once the crisis or situation passed, there was no reason to continue to engage in prostitution.[68] One colonial physician in Cameroon commented that such behavior was often the result of local chiefs using them "as a source of income,"[69] without indicating the reason for it. His comments did suggest that these women supported the income of someone who exercised authority over them.

Most of the European, Japanese, and Chinese women (if not all) who engaged in prostitution were in all probability part of the international trade in women. "International prostitution was fed by the French, the Italians, and Central European Jews (especially from Poland), together with some Russians. Above all, there were the Chinese and Japanese."[70] While initially the main route for white slavery was from Europe to Latin America, with the opening of the mines in South Africa, new routes brought white prostitutes to Africa either from New York or through the Suez Canal.[71] Hence, those white women working in Southwest Africa or Dar es Salaam most likely arrived there via this network, a fact confirmed by a DSWA police report from 1904. In that report, Sergeant Weber wrote that prostitutes were expected from South Africa on the next ship.[72] The French prostitutes working there were probably also a part of this trade because they figured prominently "in [this] global diaspora embracing Buenos Aires, the Rand [in South Africa] and Manchuria."[73] In East Africa, the widely dispersed origins of the prostitutes working in the same place in East Africa (two from Italy, five from the island of Reunion, one from the Seychelles, and two from Japan)[74] and the existing white slavery routes suggested the prominent role played by this network. The Russian prostitutes working in Qingdao were almost certainly also a part of this trade for the Russians engaged in it exported peasant women to Manchuria and northern China.[75]

The Chinese and Japanese prostitutes operating in the German overseas empire, the majority of whom worked in Qingdao and in the German Pacific territories, were often forced into prostitution through some type of contractual arrangement.[76] These contracts were usually entered into either by families or through deception. Indeed, some families escaped economic hardships by selling their daughters into prostitution and many daughters willingly went out of a sense of familial obligation. Meanwhile, other women, lured by ostensible promises of good wages, found themselves abducted and pressed into prostitution either at home or quite often overseas, such as in German New Guinea. In such situations, they often worked for a madam.[77]

In both Japan and China, most of the prostitutes came not surprisingly from the more impoverished regions. Hence, in Japan, the Japanese prostitutes (*karayuki*) came from the country's poorest region, the northern part of Kyūshū (the most southwesterly of Japan's four main islands). Chinese prostitutes generally entered into the *muti tsai* system, which essentially reduced them to servants of the people who owned their contracts. There were three types of Chinese prostitutes: sold, pawned, and volunteers. The former meant that the bordello owner kept all the earnings. A pawned woman had to work off a debt, while a volunteer received board and lodging and could keep part of her wages.[78]

Ultimately what emerged in the colonies was a situation where men continued to have access to sex, but without any apparent consequences. Of course, there were groups that opposed such a situation, primarily the missionaries who argued that men should assume responsibility for any offspring. In addition, nationalists opposed all forms of sexual encounters between the races and believed that those who crossed the lines should be excluded from the white community.[79] Yet, despite these voices of opposition, a system of mutual, even permanent, but also at times only temporary relationships was replaced by situational sex where partners were changed on a regular basis. Or, as the scholar Fatima El-Tayeb has argued, "rape and prostitution, sexual contact that is, that holds up the hierarchy and treats the black woman not as an individual, but rather as part of an anonymous, exchangeable mass, was … tolerated."[80] And, according to Hartmann, "Given the violent nature of the colonial situation … and the specific sociology of violence and sex in such situations, prostitutive forms of erotic interaction often cannot be clearly separated from coercive impositions of male sexual desire."[81]

However, such relations brought with them the chance of venereal infection. According to a doctor in Cameroon, "The real effect of domestic criticism is so far … an increase in prostitution among the natives and an increase in sexually transmitted diseases among the Europeans."[82] Like their counterparts in Germany, colonial physicians viewed the body of the prostitute and VD as synonymous. Hence, the body of the female indigene was both enticing (in that it provided an escape from the controlled, rational world of Western society) and dangerous (because it threatened that very world).[83] Consequently, female prostitutes, especially non-European ones, constituted a significant public health danger. Similar to the situation at home, physicians and their administrative supporters in the colonies focused therefore on medically regulating prostitution. From their perspective, the best way to control the spread of venereal diseases was to control the body of the prostitute. Further, prostitution was the one type of sexual contact that colonial authorities could ostensibly regulate more easily. Thus, even though men were also part of the prostitutional equation and in the context of the fight against VD were also the subject of colonial control, women in the colonies were the primary objects of regulation. The German physicians essentially saw all non-European women as prostitutes, especially but not exclusively in Africa. Along with non-European and German (primarily lower- and lower-middle-class) men, prostitutes—in particular indigenous ones—became the object of medical control. These efforts did not begin with changes to marriage laws in the colonies, but rather constituted an aspect of German colonial rule from at least the 1890s.

Nonetheless, efforts to control or at least redirect male sexuality contributed to the spread of venereal diseases in the overseas possessions. No longer did men limit themselves to a single sexual partner. Rather, they changed partners regularly, depending on the situation. And, as already noted, many of these women were seen to be carriers of VD. From the perspective of contemporaries, these diseases endangered the foundations of Germany's colonial empire. Though the response was a medical one, it contributed to the establishment and maintenance of German rule by trying to exercise greater control over those bodies deemed threatening to a colonial order based upon white, heterosexual, middle-class male values. Simultaneously, the response revealed the limitations of colonial control.

Notes

1. For example, see Luise White, *The Comforts of Home: Prostitution in Colonial Nairobi* (Chicago: University of Chicago Press, 1990), 20; Eckert, *Grundbesitz, Landkonflikte und kolonialer Wandel,* 205; Phil Bonner, "'Desirable or undesirable Basotho women?' Liquor, prostitution and migration of Basotho women to the Rand, 1920–1945," in *Women and Gender in Southern Africa to 1945,* ed. Cheryl Walker (Claremont, South Africa: David Philip Publishers, 1990), 250; Lucy Mair, *African Marriage and Social Change* (London: Frank Cass & Co., 1969), 33; Emmanuel Akyeampong, *Drink, Power, and Cultural Change. A Social History of Alcohol in Ghana c. 1900 to Recent Times* (Portsmouth, NH: Heinemann, 1996), 63; Milton Lewis and Scott Bamber, "Introduction," in *Sex, Disease, and Society: A Comparative History of Sexually Transmitted Diseases and HIV/AIDS in Asia and the Pacific,* ed. Milton Lewis, Scott Bamber, and Michael Waugh (Westport, CT: Greenwood Press, 1997), 1–17.
2. *AkG* (1899): 353.
3. The first reported presence of prostitution appeared in 1903, though it was certainly intimated in an 1894 document. See Dr. Hintze, Aerztlicher Bericht über die Zeit vom 1. Juli bis zum 30. September 03 Bezirk Lome, Togo, 29 October 1903, BArch R1001/5766, 59–60; Governor, Togo, to Colonial Department, AA, 29 October 1903, BArch R1001/5766, 58; Doering to Colonial Department, AA, 10 August 1894, BArch R1001/5765.
4. The first discovered report of prostitution was from 1902/03. *AkG* (1904): 576. However, given the nature and size of the town, it most likely existed prior to this date, similar to Lomé.
5. *MB 1905/06* (1904): 157; Jürgen Becher, *Dar es Salaam, Tanga und Tabora. Stadtentwicklung in Tansania under deutscher Kolonialherrschaft (1885–1914)* (Stuttgart: Franz Steiner, 1997), 46–47, 50; Eckert, *Grundbesitz, Landkonflikte und kolonialer Wandel,* 96, 112.
6. Dr. Richter, Krankenbericht, Windhoek, 1 November 1893, BArch R1001/5754, 16–17; *AkG* (1902–1903): 407.
7. Prostituierte im Berichtsjahre 1911/12, BArch R1001/5671, 184.
8. Liste aufgezeichneten Frauen, die auf Geschlechtskrankheiten untersucht wurden, 16 February 1914, BArch R150F/FA3/1252, 10–12; Liste der Frau in Kamina, die verdaechtig erschienen oeffentliche Maedchen zu sein, zur Untersuchung auf Geschlechtskrankheiten, 17 February

1914, BArch R150F/FA3/1252, 17; *MB 1909/10* (1911): 329; Medizinalbericht für Kamerun 1909/10, 1910, BArch R1001/6012, 1.

9. Wolfram Hartmann, "Urges in the colony: Men and women in colonial Windhoek, 1890–1914," *Journal of Namibian Studies* 1 (2007): 49–50.
10. Peter Sebald, "Das deutsche 'Fußvolk' in Togo 1884–1914," in *Transformationen der europäischen Expansion vom 16. bis zum 20. Jahrhundert. 4. Jahrestagung des Schwerpunktprogrammes der Deutschen Forschungsgemeinschaft. Forschungen zur kognitiven Interaktion europäischen Gesellschaften,* eds. Andreas Eckert and Jürgen Müller (Rehburg-Loccum: Evangelische Akademie Loccum, 1997), 178.
11. Eckart, *Medizin und Kolonialimperialismus,* 351.
12. Hartmann, "Urges in the colony," 47.
13. *MB 1911/12* (1915): 170–172; Becher, *Dar es Salaam, Tanga und Tabora,* 42.
14. Sebald, "Kolonialregime und Mischlinge," 115; Zur Ausfuehrung und genauen Kontrolle, Atakpame, 17 February 1914, BArch R150F/FA3/1252, 17; Martin Pabst, *Mission und Kolonialpolitik: Die Norddeutsche Missionsgesellschaft an der Goldküste und in Togo bis zum Ausbruck des Ersten Weltkrieges* (Munich: Anarche, 1988), 554, note 2; Regelung der Prostitution in Lome, 1908, BArch R150F/FA3/134, 98–99; Sebald, "Das deutsche 'Fußvolk,'" 178; Medizinalbericht für Kamerun 1909/10, 1910; *MB 1908/09* (1910): 511; *MB 1911/12* (1915): 420; Imperial Government, Buea, to Governor, Windhoek, 17 February 1909, BArch R151F/G.iv.D.1, 5.
15. Hartmann, "Sexual Encounters," 200.
16. *AkG* (1904): 100; Gustav Heim, "Die Syphilis in den deutschen Schutzgebieten," *Archiv für Dermatologie und Syphilis* 118 (1913): 197; Eschstruth, Polizeiverordnung, Windhoek, 25 March 1905, BArch R151F/H.ii.h.i, 83. See also John Noyes, *Colonial Space: Spatiality in the discourse of German South West Africa 1884–1915* (Chur: Harwood Academic Publishers, 1992), 272; Hartmann, "Urges in the colony," 47.
17. Hartmann, "Urges in the colony," 47.
18. Ibid., 48.
19. Seitz to RKA, 12 March 1912, BArch R1001/6010, 61–62.
20. Weber to Imperial Bezirksamt, Swakopmund, 15 October 1904, BArch R151F/G.iv.D.2, 5.
21. *AkG* (1902–03): 407.
22. Hartmann, "Urges in the colony," 49.
23. Franz Seiner, *Bergtouren und Steppenfahrten im Hererolande* (Berlin: Wilhem Süsserott, 1904), 23.
24. Hartmann, "Urges in the colony," 49–50.
25. Heim, "Die Syphilis in den deutschen Schutzgebieten," 197.
26. Hartmann, "Urges in the colony," 50–51.
27. Otto Reiner, *Achtzehn Jahre Farmer in Afrika* (Leipzig: Paul List Verlag, 1924), 41–42.
28. Bongard to Imperial Governor, 22 January 1906, BArch R151F/G.iv.D.2, 41.
29. District Officer, Grootfontein, to Imperial Government, Windhoek, 18 December 1908, BArch R151F/H.ii.H.2: 12.
30. Walther, *Creating Germans Abroad,* 57.
31. Dr. Fuchs, Imperial Bezirks Officer, Polizeiverfügung btr. das Verhalten der Prostituierten in Swakopmund, 7 September 1904, BArch R151F/G.iv.D.1, 2–4.
32. Imperial Bezirks Officers, Swakopmund, to Imperial Government, Windhoek, 7 April 1909, BArch R151F/G.iv.D.1, 6.
33. Fuchs to Imperial Police Commandant, Swakopmund, 23 December 1904, BArch R151F/G.iv.D.2, 12.
34. Fuchs, Polizeiverfügung, 7 September 1904; Imperial Bezirks Court, Swakopmund, Strafsache gegen E. Schmidt, S. Leda und A. Lebrun, 9 June 1905, BArch R151F/G.iv.D.2, 29–32.
35. Nils Oermann, *Mission, Church and State Relations in South West Africa under German Rule (1884–1915)* (Stuttgart: Franz Steiner, 1999), 212; Essner, "'Wo Rauch ist,'" 154, 156.

36. Akten des Kaiserlichen Gouvernements, State Archives, Windhoek, file W.III.f.2, cited in Noyes, *Colonial Space,* 272–273; Hartmann, "Sexual Encounters," 193–195; Hartmann, "Urges in the colony," 40, 43–45, 62; Krüger, *Kriegsbewältigung und Geschichtsbewußtsein,* 120–122; Oermann, *Mission, Church and State Relations,* 213.
37. Hyam, *Empire and Sexuality,* 139.
38. Hartmann, "Sexual Encounters," 203.
39. Ibid.; Seiner, *Bergtouren,* 165.
40. Seiner, *Bergtouren,* 165.
41. *MB 1911/12* (1915): 171, 172; *MB 1905/06* (1907): 199; *AkG* (1904): 576.
42. *MB 1905/06* (1907): 157.
43. *AkG* (1904): 624.
44. Hiery, "Germans, Pacific Islanders and Sexuality," 307. See also Stewart Firth, *New Guinea under the Germans* (Carlton: Melbourne University Press, 1983), 126; *AkG* (1904): 127.
45. *MB 1911/12* (1915): 503.
46. Davies, *Public Health and Colonialism,* 68; Firth, *New Guinea,* 117.
47. Davies, *Public Health,* 68; *MB 1911/12* (1915): 503; Hans Kersten, Aerztlicher Vierteljahresbericht für die Zeit vom 1 July–30 September 1913, BArch R1001/5772, 267; Hans Kersten, "Die Gonorrhöe im Bezirk Rabaul (Deutsch-Neuguinea)," *Beihefte zum ASTH* 29 (1925): 180–183; Kersten, Aerztlicher Vierteljahresbericht für die Zeit vom 1 January–31 March 1914, BArch R1001/5773,107.
48. Dr. Jaeschke, Vorgaenge im Kiautschou-Gebiet, 8 September 1900, Tsingtau, BArch-MA RM/6745.
49. Uthemann and Fürth, "Tsingtau," 25.
50. Annette Biener, *Das deutsche Pachtgebiet Tsingtau in Schantung, 1897–1914. Institutioneller Wandel durch Kolonialisierung* (Bonn: Matzat, 2001), 279–280; Fu-the Huang, *Qingdao: Chinesen unter deutscher Herrschaft 1897–1914* (Bochum: Projekt, 1999), 212.
51. Uthemann and Fürth, "Tsingtau," 25; Huang, *Qingdao,* 211; and Biener, *Das deutsche Pachgebiet,* 279–281.
52. Franz Kronecker, "Fünfzehn Jahre Kiautschou," *Deutsche Medizinische Presse* (1913): 16.
53. Bericht über den Gesundheitszustand des III. See-Bataillons für die Zeit vom 1 April–30 June 1913, 1 July 1913, BArch-MA, RM3/6766, 175; Wend, Hygienische Massnahmen im Bericht über den Gesundheitszustand der Matrosenartillerie-Abteilung Kiautschou für die Zeit vom 1 October–31 December 1913, 1 January 1914, BArch-MA RM3/6767, 75. See also Biener, *Das deutsche Pachgebiet,* 283.
54. Mühlhahn, *Herrschaft und Widerstand,* 259.
55. Uthemann and Fürth, "Tsingtau," 25–26; Kronecker, "Fünfzehn Jahre Kiautschou," 16. See also Huang, *Qingdao,* 211–212; Kersten, Aerztlicher Vierteljahresbericht für 1 January–31 March 1914, 1914.
56. Sitzung des Bezirksbeirats Keetmanshoop, 21 November 1908, BAarch R151F/G.iv.D.2, 77d–77e.
57. Peter Sack and Dymphna Clark, ed., *German New Guinea: The Annual Reports* (Canberra: Australian National University Press, 1979), 267.
58. Thoralf Klein, "Rasse—Kultur—soziale Stellung: Konzeptionen des 'Eingeborenen' und koloniale Segregation in Kiautschou," in *Rassenmischehen,* 304–328; Pabst, *Mission and Kolonialpolitik,* 554, especially note 2.
59. Although the author discusses the situation in Australia, it applies equally well to other colonial situations. Raelene Davidson, "'As good a bloody woman as any other woman …': Prostitutes in Western Australia, 1895–1939," in *Exploring Women's Pasts: Essays in Social History,* ed. Patricia Crawford et al. (London: Allen & Unwin, 1984 [1983]), 190–191.
60. For example, see Charles van Onselen, *Studies in the Social and Economic History of Witwatersrand 1886–1914,* vol. I, *New Babylon* (New York: Longman, 1982), 108ff.; Raelene Fran-

ces, "Sex Workers or Citizens? Prostitution and the Shaping of 'Settler' Society in Australia," *International Review of Social History* 44 (1999): 101–122.

61. White, *The Comforts of Home,* 1–2, 48–50.
62. Belinda Bozzoli, *Women of Phokeng: Consciousness, Life Strategy, and Migrancy in South Africa, 1900–1933* (Portsmouth, NH: Heinemann, 1991), 81, 91; Mair, *African Marriage,* 43, 55, 65, 141; Kenneth Little, *African Women in Towns: An Aspect of Africa's Social Revolution* (Cambridge: Cambridge University Press, 1973), 76.
63. Seiner, *Bergtouren,* 165.
64. Hartmann, "Urges in the colony," 62.
65. White, *Comforts of Home,* 1, 15, 37; Mair, *African Marriage,* 55–65.
66. Medizinalbericht für Kamerun 1909/10, 1910.
67. Sitzung des Bezirksbeirats Keetmanshoop, 21 November 1908.
68. Mair, *African Marriage,* 141, 147, 43; White, *Comforts of Home,* 20, 34.
69. *AkG* (1904): 576
70. Hyam, *Empire and Sexuality,* 142.
71. Ibid., 45, 148.
72. Weber to Imperial Bezirksamt, Swakopmund, 15 October 1904, BArch R151F/G.iv.D.2, 5. For a more detailed account of prostitution in South Africa, see van Onselen, *Social and Economic History of Witwatersrand,* 103–162.
73. Hyam, *Empire and Sexuality,* 146.
74. *MB 1911/12* (1915): 170.
75. Hyam, *Empire and Sexuality,* 144–145.
76. Ibid., 140.
77. Gail Hershatter, *Dangerous Pleasures: Prostitution and Modernity in Twentieth-Century Shanghai* (Berkeley: University of California Press, 1997), 182, 191; D. C. S. Sissons, "*Karayuki-san*: Japanese Prostitutes in Australia, 1887–1916—I," *Historical Studies* 17 (1977): 323–341; Christian Henriot, *Prostitution and Sexuality in Shanghai: A Social History, 1849–1949,* trans. Noël Castelino (Cambridge: Cambridge University Press, 2001), 185, 188–191.
78. Hyam, *Empire and Sexuality,* 140.
79. Sebald, "Kolonialregime und Mischlinge," 115; Walther, *Creating Germans Abroad,* 39–41.
80. El-Tayeb, "Verbotene Begegnungen," 90.
81. Although he writes specifically about DSWA, I would argue that his comments apply to all German colonies. Hartmann, "Sexual Encounters," 187.
82. *MB 1907/08* (1909): 200–201. See also Walther, "Sex, Race and Empire," 45–71.
83. Spongberg, *Feminizing Venereal Disease,* 6, 35; Gilman, *Difference and Pathology,* 94; Schulte, *Sperrbezirke,* 7, 35; Ulrich, "Ärzte und Sexualität," 223–235, 229; and Gilman, "Black Sexuality and Modern Consciousness," 50.

PART II

Venereal Disease in the Colonial Context

Chapter 4

THE THREAT OF VENEREAL DISEASE

Within the context of colonial public health, numerous diseases posed a serious threat to the establishment and maintenance of German control over its colonial possessions, such as malaria and sleeping sickness.[1] However, none was perceived to be as universally threatening as venereal diseases to the foundations of German colonialism. Across all the colonies and throughout the period of German rule, colonial doctors repeatedly spoke of how widespread and dangerous VD was. For instance, Dr. Schwabe noted that in the mid-1890s "there is not a disease … that has the same significance as syphilis" among the native population on Jaluit in German New Guinea.[2] In the early 1900s, Dr. Krüger reported that in Lomé, Togo, VD accounted for "the second highest percentage of the illnesses" behind malaria among Europeans.[3] In Cameroon, Dr. Heuermann believed that "50 percent of all local Europeans [were] smitten by venereal diseases."[4] Even in 1911/12, Dr. Meixner, the chief medical officer for the East African Imperial Troops (*kaiserliche Schutztruppe*), reported that "venereal diseases still entail a noteworthy increase among the colored military personnel."[5] The concern over venereal diseases was closely tied to the vitality and future of the German overseas empire. There were three areas of anxiety for colonial authorities: military effectiveness, economic vitality, and the health of the white ruling elite.

Similar to the situation in Germany and in other European colonies,[6] physicians in the overseas territories noted that venereal diseases reduced the fighting capacity of regular and colonial (both indigenous and German) military forces. According to the scholar Douglas Peers, armies constituted "the ultimate expression of colonial rule."[7] This was especially true during the Maji Maji War in East Africa and the Nama and Herero Wars in DSWA (1904–1907). During the latter

Notes for this section begin on page 56.

conflict, a Southwest African Health Office complained that the spread of VD "severely damaged the health and readiness of the colonial troops."[8] Moreover, the annual medical reports provided statistical evidence of the reduction in the efficacy of colonial soldiers. For example, in 1907/08, 531 cases of gonorrhea were treated for 14,924 days and 117 were treated for constitutional syphilis for 2,800 days.[9]

Similar reports existed for other colonies, where the number of cases and the days treated were reported assiduously. For instance, in Cameroon among the "colored" (*Farbige*) colonial troops, there were 419 cases of VD for the year 1900/01, 248 of which were new incidents of gonorrhea, each of which was treated for an average of 17.9 days. Each of the 27 new cases of syphilis was treated for an average of 42 days.[10] Meanwhile, as early as 1893 in DSWA, Dr. Richter stated that after his "weekly examination of the [white] soldiers for venereal diseases would lead to nearly all the 300-man troop being sent to the military hospital or least a large percentage of them, so that the purpose of the force would be impaired."[11]

Further, colonial authorities pointed out that sexually transmitted diseases lowered the productive function of the indigenous workforce, thus undermining the potential economic output of the colony and the empire as a whole. Similar fears existed in other European colonies.[12] In Germany's possessions, recorded figures indicated that VD was having an impact on the labor force. For instance, from July 1898 to June 1899, the New Guinea annual report indicated that venereal diseases accounted for 8,222 sick days (i.e., work days lost), or nearly 36 percent of the total among the indigenous workforce.[13] In Cameroon, one physician in Dume reported that in 1909/10 "the largest group that misses work regularly are from those infected with venereal disease."[14]

According to Hans Ziemann, a longtime physician in Africa, "what good are an abundance of colonial goods …, if there are not enough natives to harvest them, or if through laziness they let them fall to ruin."[15] For Ludwig Külz, "the people" possessed "colonial economic capital value" (*kolonialwirtschaftlicher Kapitalswert*), not just "our colonial mineral resources, forestry, and livestock." As a matter of fact, he viewed indigenes as "the most valuable colonial possession."[16]

The spread of VD among indigenous populations was closely tied to the concern over falling birthrates in the Pacific and Africa.[17] In the early years of the twentieth century, reports from the island territories in German New Guinea raised fears among colonial authorities about the ostensible decline in the indigenous populations, a situation that would undermine the economic viability of the colonies in the future. As early as 1901, Dr. Sunder wrote about "the decline of the brown inhabitants of Yap [in the Caroline Islands]." He stated that it "would be a shame if this nice, lovable, willing to work, culturally high standing people would belong to the past." For him, the causes were "tuberculosis, syphilis, [and] gonorrhea" as well as "moral and social conditions."[18] More than a decade later, Dr. Born expressed similar concerns about the population on the Ebon Atoll in the Marshall Islands, writing that gonorrhea "exercises a harmful influence on the ability of both sexes to reproduce."[19] His colleague on the atoll of Jaluit in the Marshalls, Dr. Karl Kopp, identified syphilis as a reason for the reduction in the population.[20]

Similarly, officials in Africa expressed anxiety over the impact venereal diseases had on the indigenous population. For instance, Governor Bruno von Schuckmann (1907–1910) in DSWA informed the Imperial Colonial Office in early 1908 that VD threatened the preservation (*Erhaltung*) "of the black worker population."[21] This apprehension appeared again later that year in the memorandum intended to combat this threat. In the document, it was noted that "such a contamination of the native population with venereal diseases poses a great danger for the economic development of the protectorate, because these diseases severely endanger the healthy offspring (*Nachwuchs*) of the urgently necessary worker population."[22]

In Cameroon, medical officials reported that venereal diseases among indigenous adults contributed to "a gradually progressive degeneration of the offspring,"[23] which would undermine the economic development of the colony.[24] Dr. Ernst Rodenwaldt attributed the apparent population decline among the Akposso in Togo in part to the "decreased fertility among women which" was the result of "an increase in venereal disease brought on by the dislocations of colonial rule."[25] In German East Africa, there were also worries about the death rate among children. A longtime settler in the colony, Baron von Dalwigk, contended that VD spread through prostitution threatened to reduce significantly the autochthonous population.[26] However, Governor Heinrich Schnee disputed Dalwigk's assertion, noting that the death rate among children was more likely due to other factors, such as "deficiencies in children's nutrition, epidemics, … [and] migrant labor."[27] Some doctors, though, did attribute a low birth rate to VD, but increasingly more and more concluded "among most African peoples [there], the birth rate was moderate" in part as a result of "traditional methods of birth control."[28]

In reality, though, evidence from today demonstrates that even if the populations were declining, it was not as severe as contemporaries believed. As Stewart Firth explains in his study of German New Guinea, "In societies where women and children frequently fled into the bush at the approach of Europeans, census takers could be misled into underestimating the number of inhabitants and producing spurious exact statistics revealing the depopulation which they expected to find. German censuses in New Guinea were no exception and must have been considerably distorted by the fact that the district officer who came to count the people also came to collect the tax."[29]

Moreover, contemporary observers were often wrong in their assessment of the causes. This could have been a result of their unwillingness to examine the real reasons because this would have resulted in a criticism of German colonialism.[30] The reasons given by Governor Schnee were perhaps among the most accurate assessments. At any rate, regardless of the demographic truth, contemporaries believed that venereal diseases contributed not only to a drop in the productive function of the indigenous labor force at the moment, but also to a reduction in the potential labor pool in the future.[31]

Finally, in some locations, health officials reported that venereal diseases threatened the hegemonic role played by whites, now and in the future. Dr. Heim remarked that in the South Seas, "the infected native population is a terrible source of infection for Europeans."[32] In DSWA, Germany's primary settler colony, one doctor expressed his surprise that entire white families were not infected because so many diseased "native" servant women worked in white households. "There were some venereal diseased people (*Geschlechtskranke*), whose illness was so disgusting and neglected, that you must call it a miracle if their employers' families were not infected. If one looks at how these patients handle their sores and then with the contaminated fingers touch without delay tableware, utensils, etc ... , so the possibility of the non-sexual infection is no longer small. The contamination of the Windhoek natives with syphilis will reach in a short time such a degree that it will have serious consequences for the white population."[33] Indeed, the situation was so serious that Governor Seitz in 1911 reported to the Imperial Colonial Office (RKA) in Berlin that venereal diseases "considerably made more difficult the settlement of the country" and will be "of serious consequences both for the ability to propagate and for healthy descendants of the whites."[34] Similar concerns existed in other European colonies, especially those with larger white populations such as South Africa and Rhodesia (present-day Zimbabwe).[35]

Notes

1. Eckart, *Medizin und Kolonialimperialismus*; Isobe, *Medizin und Kolonialgesellschaft.*
2. *AkG* (1897): 74.
3. *AkG* (1904): 584, 585.
4. *MB 1905/06* (1907): 389.
5. *MB 1911/12* (1915): 630.
6. Levine, *Prostitution, Race and Politics,* 57–59, 111, 123–124, 267–269.
7. Though he writes about British India, his remarks apply equally well to all colonial situations, including the German. Douglas Peers, "Contours of the Garrison State: The Army and the Historiography of Early Nineteenth-Century India," in *Orientalism, Evangelicalism and the Military Cantonment in Early Nineteenth-Century India: A Historiographical Overview,* ed. Nancy Cassels (Lewiston: Edwin Mellon Press, 1991), 90.
8. Medical Office, DSWA, Denkschrift zur Bekämpfung der Geschlechtskrankheiten im Südwestafrikanischen Schutzgebiet, 5 November 1908, BArch R1001/6040, 17.
9. *MB 1907/08* (1909): 311.
10. *AkG* (1904): 73, 74.
11. Richter, Krankenbreicht, Windhoek, 1 November 1893, BArch R1001/5754, 16–18.
12. Philip Setel, "Comparative Histories of Sexually Transmitted Diseases and HIV/AIDS in Africa: An Introduction," in *Histories of Sexually Transmitted Diseases and HIV/AIDS in Sub-Saharan Africa,* ed. Philip Setel, Milton Lewis, and Maryinez Lyons (Westport, CT: Greenwood Press, 1999), 3; Karen Jochelson, "Sexually Transmitted Diseases in Nineteenth- and Twentieth-Century South Africa," in *Histories of Sexually Transmitted Diseases,* 230.

13. Sack and Clark, *German New Guinea,* 159.
14. *MB 1909/10* (1911): 328.
15. Hans Ziemann, "Wie erobert man Afrika für die weiße und farbige Rasse?" *Beiheft zum ASTH* 11, no. 5 (1907), 7.
16. Ludwig Külz, "Grundzüge der kolonialen Eingeborenenhygiene," *Beiheft zum ASTH* 15 (1911): 14–15, 18.
17. Eckart, *Medizin und Kolonialimperialismus,* 437–440; Davies, *Public Health and Colonialism,* 154–174; Koponen, *Development for Exploitation,* 495–499, 585–605; Rudin, *Germans in the Cameroons,* 345–353.
18. Dr. Sunder, Krankheiten auf Yap, 12 April 1901, BArch R1001/5775, 42.
19. Dr. Born, Die gesundheitliche Verhältnisse auf dem Atoll Ebon, November 1913, BArch R1001/5788, 30.
20. Kopp to RKA State Secretary, 23 August 1913, NAA/G2/U24, 22–25.
21. Bruno to RKA, 8 January 1908, BArch R1001/6040, 3.
22. Medical Office, DSWA, Denkschrift zur Bekämpfung der Geschlechtskrankheiten, 5 November 1908, 15–16.
23. *MB 1909/10* (1911): 328.
24. Denkchrift über die weitere Entwicklung des Gesundheitswesens in Kamerun, 1913, BArch R1001/5764, 5–9.
25. Arthur Knoll, *Togo under Imperial Germany 1884–1914* (Stanford, CA: Hoover Institution Press, 1978), 91.
26. Baron von Dalwigk, Der Geburtenrückgang und die Kindersterblichkeit in Deutsch-Ostafrika infolge der Prostitution und der durch dieselbe entstandenen Krankheiten, BArch R1001/5671, 145–153.
27. Schnee to State Secretary, RKA, 14 June 1913, BArch R1001/5671, 182.
28. Koponen, *Development for Exploitation,* 498–499. See also Eckart, *Medizin und Kolonialimperialismus,* 313.
29. Firth, *New Guinea,* 113.
30. Wolfgang Eckart, "Medicine and German colonial expansion in the Pacific: the Caroline, Mariana, and Marshall Islands," in *Disease, Medicine, and Empire: Perspectives on Western Medicine and the Experience of European Expansion,* ed. Roy Macleod and Milton Lewis (London: Routledge, 1988), 85–91.
31. Davies, *Public Health and Colonialism*, 4; Grosse, *Kolonialismus, Eugenik und bügerliche Gesellschaft,* 114. Grosse also suggests that part of the effort to prevent the extermination of indigenous populations was to minimize their proletarianization, though he provides no supporting evidence.
32. Heim, "Die Syphilis in den deutschen Schutzgebieten," 196.
33. Stabarzt, Report to Sanitation Office, Windhoek, 1910, BArch R151F/H.ii.h.i, 74.
34. Seitz to RKA, 24 September 1911, BArch R1001/6042, 70.
35. Jochelson, "Sexually Transmitted Diseases," 230; Jock McCulloch, "The Management of Venereal Disease in Settler Society: Colonial Zimbabwe, 1900–30," in *Histories of Sexually Transmitted Diseases,* 198.

Chapter 5

ASSESSING THE THREAT STATISTICALLY

Concerns about the spread of venereal diseases were based largely on the statistical data collected by colonial doctors. As in Germany, statistics became a means of surveillance that was used to evaluate the health of the colonies and to identify threats to it. The collection of this data was part of the larger phenomenon of gathering statistical information to assess the efficacy of German colonialism. However, the compiling of data also provided "an instrument for regulating and transforming" colonial populations, especially through the act of classification.[1]

One of the primary vehicles for this was the annual reports for each colony. In terms of total number of pages, a significant portion of them consisted of statistics. The data collected included information on the population, including figures for men, women, and children according to racial categories, birth and death rates, professions, country of origin, etc. Other entries provided information on the economy, which included sections on production, trade, and transportation, and finances, which focused mainly on each colony's income and expenses. In the population reports, colonial inhabitants were divided primarily into two categories: "white" (*weiße*) and "colored" (*farbige*), although subcategories of the latter included "colored, indigenes" (*farbige, Eingegorene*), "colored, non-indigenes" (*farbige, Nichteingeborene*) and "mestee" (*Mischlinge*).[2]

Colonial doctors also collected data and contributed to the categorization of the colonial population in their regular medical reports on the health situation in the various overseas territories. These reports were published as an addendum to the annual colonial report to the Reichstag and in various other periodicals. In order to centralize the dissemination of "experiences scientifically gained in the colonies," the Imperial Health Office in 1897, at the request of the Colonial

Notes for this section begin on page 73.

Office, began publishing them in the *Arbeiten des Kaiserlichen Gesundheitsamte* (Publication of the Imperial Health Office).[3] Starting in 1905, the Colonial Department of the German Foreign Office, then later the Imperial Colonial Office, published annually all colonial medical reports in its own periodical, *Medizinal-Berichte über die Deutschen Schutzgebiete.*

In the collection of statistical data, colonial physicians contributed to the colonial enterprise in several ways. On the surface, their purpose was to provide a summary of the overall health of each colony. For instance, the 1909/10 record for German East Africa (present-day Tanzania) included nineteen different statistical appendices on such subjects as the number of immunizations, of ill (*kranke*) "Europeans" (*Europäer*) and "coloreds" (*Farbige*), of Europeans who died, of blood examinations for malaria, and of rat exterminations.[4] Similar to the metropole,[5] such information could reveal the efficacy of various policies or indicate where new or additional steps needed to be taken in order to protect or promote the public health in the colony.

With regards to the sick or diseased (*kranke*), data was systematically entered. For instance, in the appendices for "Europeans" and "coloreds," VD was usually category VII, with each specific venereal illness often having its own number. For each specific disease, patients were usually described numerically in three different ways. The first category was "treated." The next was the outcome of that treatment: "healed," "died," "elsewhere," or "continuing." The final category indicated the number of days that they had been in treatment either in a hospital or in a clinic (though the last two reporting years, 1910/11 and 1911/12, did not use this category in the tables). Thus, each patient was reduced to a numerical aggregate and in essence became a "thing" to be acted upon—e.g., "treated" and eventually "healed." Moreover, the impact of the treatment was measured in the number of days that they were not active in society (i.e., not contributing to the colonial endeavor).[6]

As in Germany, the collection of data in the colonies was problematic at best and only provided a limited view of the actual health of the colonies. Notwithstanding, physicians in Africa interpreted the numbers as an indication of the prevalence of venereal diseases among the colonial populations, including whites. In Cameroon, for instance, physicians noted a steady increase in the number of cases in Douala over the years. In the other two main districts, Victoria and Kribi, there were initially very few cases and, though the numbers rose over time, by 1909/10 there was a noticeable decline. When looking at the entire colony, though, the amount increased. In 1903/04, there were only 7 recorded cases. By 1911/12, the total number of reported cases had risen to 154. This was 8.5 percent of the colony's European population[7] and more than double the previous year's count of 71 (see appendix, tables 3–4).

Compared to other infectious diseases, VD had become one of the most common illnesses in the colony by 1911/12. In that year, 154 of the reported cases for Europeans (out of a total of 671) were for VD or 23 percent of all reported cases. In terms of sheer numbers, venereal infections as a whole were second only behind malaria (166 cases) in 1911/12. In fact, bubo was the second most frequent infectious disease that year (84) and syphilis was third (69). Dysentery came in fourth with 44 incidents and gonorrhea fifth with 38.[8]

Moreover, in terms of the average number of treatment days, venereal diseases were one of the highest among contagious diseases. In 1903/04, the figure was 16.4 days for whites. Dysentery averaged 10.3 days (8 patients for 82 days), while malaria had only an average treatment of 6.8 days (135 patients for a total of 916 days) and black water fever an average of 7.3 days (26 patients for 190 days). By 1909/10 (the last year treatment days for individual illnesses were provided), VD continued to have one of the highest averages of days treated. For whites, the figure had dropped by just over 2 to 13.7 days. Broken down by specific venereal infections, this meant that on average Europeans were treated 12.3 days for gonorrhea (24 patients for 295 days) and 16 for syphilis (15 cases for 240 days). By comparison, each white patient was treated an average of 7.3 days for malaria (186 patients for 1362 days), 14.9 for black water fever (38 cases for 566 days), and 19 days for dysentery (38 patients for 609 days).[9] Thus, VD as a whole fell behind black water fever and dysentery, but syphilis still had the second highest average.

On the opposite coast, in German East Africa, venereal diseases were also spreading and rising in frequency among Europeans. In fact, one medical official described them as a "pestilence."[10] The number grew from 79 in 1903/04 to 276 in 1911/12 (the high point was 302 in 1910/11), or by more than three times (see appendix, table 9). As in Cameroon, larger urban centers had more VD patients than rural areas. For example, in Dar es Salaam, the colony's largest town, VD was also on the rise among both Europeans and Africans. In 1903/04, there were 14 reported cases there, or nearly one-fifth of the entire colony. In 1911/12, the number had grown to 104, or nearly one-third of all cases (see appendix, table 11).

When compared to other diseases, venereal diseases occupied a significant position in the colony's public health. The 1903/04 report revealed that there were only 77 cases of VD compared to malaria, which had the most cases (298). Black water fever had 34 patients. As a percentage, VD accounted for 8.5 percent of all patients registered. As a percentage of the population, the number was slightly less, just under 7 percent (79 out of 1,200). When looking at the number of treatment days, VD accounted for 9 percent of all white patients treated in a hospital (340 out of 3,780) and 20 percent of all treated in a clinic (1,245 out of 6,370), or the second largest category for both types of facilities. However, an examination of the average number of treatment days/patients revealed that venereal diseases were the highest of all categories with 20.1 days/patient. By 1911/12, VD was still one of the largest categories, but it only had one-fifth of the malaria numbers. In terms of all patients for that year, just over 6 percent were infected with a venereal disease.[11] In terms of the European population as a whole, the percentage had fallen to approximately 5.7 percent.[12]

Although the reports were irregular, most likely as a result of the wars in the colony,[13] venereal infections in Southwest Africa were also prominent. In 1908,

Governor Seitz referred to VD as a "contamination" in the colony.[14] In 1902/03, 102 cases were reported, which, according to Dr. Hummel, was "the highest percentage among all diseases with 19.8 percent."[15] By 1907/08, the number had more than doubled, with 256 patients treated. The following year's report indicated that there was an increase in the number of VD cases (336). This meant that about 3 percent of the white population (11,791) suffered from venereal infections. The 1910/11 report indicated that the number had risen to 384, or almost 4 percent of all Europeans (10,456).[16]

Within the context of public health, venereal infections had an important impact on the white population. In 1907/08, VD (with 256 patients) was also behind infectious and general diseases (471), or 12 percent of all new patients (2,198). In terms of days treated, venereal infections were second (3,970) behind the infectious and general diseases (5,899), or 20.7 percent of the total treatment days. The most common disease was intestinal catarrh (171), then the flu (155), malaria (101), syphilis (97), dysentery (88), and finally gonorrhea (80). Three years later in 1910/11, venereal diseases were still one of the more prominent illnesses. As a group, they were the third largest (384) behind infectious and general illnesses (737) or 9 percent of all new illnesses (4,137), a drop of 3 percent since 1907/08, but an increase of 128 actual venereal patients (384 compared to 256 in 1907/08). In terms of specific diseases, the most frequently recorded contagious illnesses were first malaria (233), then syphilis (201), and gonorrhea (137).[17]

In Togo, the situation was slightly different. Like the other colonies, venereal diseases spread throughout the colony and initially grew in frequency. According to the tabulated information, it appeared that from 1907/08 onward, VD infections were increasing, reaching a highpoint two years later in 1909/10 with 127 reported cases. In two districts that year, at least 40 percent of the white population suffered from VD. For example, in Lomé the local doctor treated 97 Europeans out of a population of 205, or about 47 percent of the population, while his colleague in Anecho reported that 18 of the 46 Europeans were treated for VD, or 40 percent. However, unlike the other African territories, by 1911/12, the last reporting year, venereal diseases appeared to be on the decline with only 85 reported for the entire colony (see appendix, tables 1–2). Nonetheless, when compared with other illnesses, venereal diseases remained prominent throughout the colonial period. In 1911/12, venereal diseases in Togo accounted for 16.7 percent of all illnesses. Moreover, among infectious diseases, VD was second behind malaria (with 95 cases) and ahead of dysentery (with 51).[18]

The prevalence of VD among military personnel in Africa was uneven, though indigenous soldiers generally experienced higher infection rates than the German soldiers. Nevertheless, in Southwest Africa German colonial troops had one of the highest morbidity rates among white colonial soldiers. One of the earliest reports of VD in DSWA came from Chief Military Physician Dr. Richter in 1893, which indicated that sexually transmitted diseases were widespread among white military personnel.[19] Apparently after the onset of the 1904–1907 Herero and Nama Wars, which also witnessed a significant increase in German troops in the colony, the incidents of VD also rose. Chief Medical Officer Dr. Schelle noted in his 1906/07 report, "Most remarkable was the strong increase in venereal disease among the troops. It was apparently connected to the increase of prisoners and movement of natives from the field."[20] The following year, there were 760 new cases of VD out of a total of 4950, or 15 percent. Moreover, treatment days for venereal diseases amounted to 19,440 (out of 68,629) or 28 percent of the total[21] (see also appendix, table 8).

In contrast, venereal diseases were infrequent among German colonial soldiers in East Africa. Throughout the colonial period, the number of infected remained largely in the single digits, except for the mid-1890s, when the colonial army was relatively new. In those years, the figures were in the double digits going as high as seventeen, but dropped by more than half after 1896/97. In 1906/07, the number rose again into the double digits to eleven, only to fall significantly the following year. In that year, venereal diseases only accounted for 1.5 percent of total troop strength, a sharp drop from the previous year's 5.7 percent, or the 6.5 percent in 1904/05. In the years after 1906/07, there were no reports of VD in published accounts (see appendix, table 12), which either meant that there was none or was statistically insignificant.

In Cameroon, venereal diseases among white colonial soldiers were practically nonexistent. The greatest number reported was six in 1908/09. In many years, though, military doctors recorded no infections after their periodic health inspections (see appendix, table 5). Dr. Heuermann remarked in 1901/02 report that "it is striking that no sexually transmitted diseases are listed, but my previous experiences have led me to the certainty that the colony is strongly contaminated with both gonorrhea and syphilis."[22]

However, regarding indigenous soldiers, military physicians in Cameroon saw venereal diseases as especially threatening. Though apparently still common in the final reporting years—one doctor noted in 1911/12 that sexually transmitted diseases were "predominant"[23]—they were nonetheless not as frequent as in the earlier reports from 1900/01 and 1901/02. In those early years, VD accounted for over 40 percent of the troop strength. In subsequent years, the numbers fell mainly into the twentieth percentile range. The rate was consistently higher than that for the civilian population, both European and African, at least until almost near the end of German colonial rule (see appendix, table 5).

With regard to the African colonial soldiers in East Africa, the Askari,[24] venereal diseases were extremely prevalent and on the rise in terms of total numbers. For instance, in 1894/95, 400 cases were reported and by 1911/12, 853 were. The most recorded number of cases was in 1910/11 with 951, but the previous year witnessed the lowest number (339). But, even as a percentage of troop strength and total number of new cases, VD had a significant presence. In 1903/04, 41 percent of the Askari were infected with a venereal disease. After that the percentage started to fall, but still remained in the twentieth percentile. In fact, in the last reported year (1911/12), VD still accounted for 28 percent of troop strength and 17.4 percent of all new treated illnesses (see appendix, table 12).

Among civilian indigenes, venereal diseases were generally more common and growing at a faster rate than among whites. For example, in East Africa, the number of infected increased steadily during the period between 1903/04 and 1911/12 from 996 reported cases to 2,650 or by 2.7 times (see appendix, table 9). When compared to other diseases, VD played a prominent role. For example, in 1903/04 among infectious diseases, venereal diseases were second in significance. In fact, there were more VD patients (996) than malaria (701). As a percentage of all illnesses, they accounted for almost 9 percent (996 out of 11,145). In terms of treatment days, 35 percent of all those treated in a hospital (17,399 out of 49,356) and nearly 7 percent of those who went to the clinic (7,774 out of 115,342) were infected with VD. As an average, this amounted to 25.3 days/patient, higher than any other category. In 1911/12, the number of VD cases had grown to 2,650, placing them third behind malaria (3,584) and sleeping sickness (5,352) among the contagious diseases. As a percentage of all patients, the number had fallen to 5 percent, but the overall number of recorded ailments had also grown to more than 4.5 times the 1903/04 figure (to 51,624 cases).[25] From the perspective of the colonial government, VD was still "widespread" in the colony in 1913. Governor Schnee, in a letter to the Colonial Office, remarked that he did not "underestimate the importance of combating venereal diseases among the colored population."[26]

With regard to the "colored" population, venereal diseases in Togo appeared to be on the rise and their numbers were larger than those experienced by whites. The highest number reported was 362 cases in 1908/09. Over the following two years there was a decrease, but they rose again in 1911/12 to 311 (see appendix, table 1). In comparison to other diseases, VD was not as prevalent as other contagious diseases. For instance, in 1905/06 the local physician's report in Lomé indicated that gonorrhea was the fourth largest infectious disease (45 cases) behind dysentery (70) and malaria (113), or just under 2 percent of all patients (45 out of 2,502). In 1911/12, a group of indigenes treated for a venereal disease (202) in the capital ranked far behind transmittable and general illnesses (the largest with 650 cases), like malaria (248 patients) and smallpox (with 159 cases). Hence, out of all the illnesses treated (3,907), VD accounted for a little more than 5 percent. In Anecho that same year, the numbers were even less, similar to the situation with Europeans there. In 1911/12, venereal diseases amounted to 65 out of a total of 1,916 patients, or 3 percent of all reported cases.[27] Nonetheless, they were still seen as a public health threat because of their persistence and impact on the labor force and white community.

In Cameroon, incidents of VD were increasing among the indigenous population. In 1903/04, physicians reported 43 cases, while in 1911/12 doctors began treating 1,105 indigenes (156 fewer than the previous year's high of 1,261). In 1907/08 Douala and Victoria, the number of cases among Africans jumped to 118 (from 82 the previous year) and 158 (from 32 in 1906/07) respectively, indicating a sharp spike in VD over previous years. There was, though, a marked decline in Kribi that year. Moreover, in general the number of reported cases fell over subsequent years in these main areas even though venereal infections were rising in the territory as a whole (see appendix, tables 3 and 4).

Compared to whites, the percentage of VD infection was lower among Africans, but it was nonetheless significant. In 1911/12, for example, VD accounted for 13 percent (or 1,105 out of a total of 8,453) of the total number of indigenes in treatment, for whites it was nearly 20 percent (154 out of 780). However, among infectious diseases in terms of absolute numbers, gonorrhea had the most patients (543), second was malaria (498), third dysentery (341), and fourth syphilis (319). Moreover, through the lens of average number of treatment days, venereal diseases were the highest among contagious diseases. In 1909/10, the average number of treatment days was 21.5. Gonorrhea averaged 22.1 (446 patients for 9837 days), syphilis 26.7 (175 cases for 4663 days), ulcus molle 16.2 (75 patients for 1218 days), and bubo 15.7 days (84 cases for 1315 days). Meanwhile, malaria had an average of 4.7 days (287 patients for 1345 days), smallpox 31.2 (23 cases for 718 days), and dysentery 14 (291 patients for 4065 days).[28] Apart from the smallpox outbreak, venereal diseases collectively and even individually therefore had the highest average number of treatment days among sick indigenes.

Venereal diseases were also apparently widespread among the indigenous population of SWA. In 1902/03, there were 408 cases, which accounted for 31.6 percent of all diseases that year. Four years later, the number had dropped to 360, but in subsequent years there was a near steady rise. For example, in 1907/08, the number stood at 470, but in the following year there was a slight drop to 463. However, by 1910/11, the number of cases had increased to 700 (see appendix, table 6). This meant that in 1907/08, VD cases accounted for 25.5 percent of all treated Africans (1,843) and for 30 percent of the total number of treatment days (13,168 out of 43,708). The following year, 29 percent of all cases (463 out of 1,578) and a staggering 58 percent of the treatment days (13,570 out of 23,358) were attributed to venereal patients. This corresponded roughly to only 0.7 percent of the estimated African population (63,117). By 1910/11, even though the absolute number of infections had increased, VD accounted for 22 percent of the cases (out of 3,142), or 7 percent less than in 1908/09. According to the census for that year in twelve districts, this amounted to 2 percent of the African population (33,344).[29] Hence, while the absolute numbers were high, as a percentage of the population the frequency of VD was low.

Compared to other diseases in SWA, venereal infections were prominent, either in terms of individual diseases or as a group. Among Africans in 1910/11, VD occupied second place (700) behind contagious and general illnesses (805), or 22.3 percent of all new ailments (3,142). That year, syphilis was by far the most common illness among all the reported cases (399) and gonorrhea was third (229). Scurvy was the second most frequent with 274.[30]

In Africa, various types of venereal diseases were present. However, gonorrhea and syphilis were consistently the most common. In Togo, for example, these two diseases consistently accounted for at least two-thirds of the cases reported among both Europeans and indigenes. Gonorrhea, though, was the most prevalent, amounting sometimes by itself to half or even two-thirds of the total number of cases treated. For instance, among whites in 1909/10, 72 of the 127 cases reported were gonorrhea (57 percent), while in 1910/11, there were 70 cases of gonorrhea out of a total of 118 VD patients (59 percent). Meanwhile, for Africans, gonorrhea cases accounted for 61 percent (1909/10), 52 percent (1910/11), and 59 percent (1911/12) of all VD patients (see appendix, table 2).

In Cameroon, gonorrhea and syphilis were also usually the most frequent venereal diseases among whites. Initially, there were just as many cases or more of gonorrhea as there were of syphilis among Europeans. However, by 1911/12, more whites were diagnosed with syphilis than gonorrhea, with 28 reported cases of gonorrhea compared to 69 cases of syphilis. In that year, though, syphilis fell behind bubo (84) as the venereal disease with the most recorded patients. The previous year 27 whites were treated for gonorrhea compared to 18 for syphilis and 18 for bubo (see Table 4).

Gonorrhea and syphilis were also apparently widespread among the indigenous Cameroonian population, though bubo and ulcus molle were frequent as well. Indeed, over the years, similar to Europeans, the number of Africans diagnosed with syphilis and gonorrhea rose. In 1903/04, there were 23 cases of gonorrhea and four with syphilis. By 1911/12, doctors reported 543 gonorrhea and 319 syphilis cases. The previous year represented the greatest number for these illnesses, with physicians treating 649 gonorrheal and 401 syphilitic patients. Cases of ulcus molle and bubo also increased over the years. In 1903/04, doctors reported 9 patients with ulcus molle and 7 with bubo, while in 1911/12 they recorded 129 of the former and 98 of the later (see appendix, table 4).

The most common venereal diseases in Southwest Africa were also gonorrhea and syphilis. Indeed, while other diseases were present, gonorrhea and syphilis consistently accounted for the overwhelming majority of venereal infections among white civilians and Africans as well as colonial soldiers. In 1907/08, for example, 70 percent of all venereal disease patients within the colonial army (531 out of 758) suffered from gonorrhea. For syphilis the amount was a little over 15 percent of all VD cases (117 out of 758). From the available data, it also appeared that gonorrhea was initially the main venereal illness among Africans. For instance, in 1907/08 and 1908/09, the percentage of VD patients with gonorrhea was 63 percent (297 out of 470) and 48 percent (221 out of 463) respectively. However, by 1910/11, syphilis had surpassed gonorrhea as the more frequent illness within the African population. In 1907/08, syphilis accounted for 31.7 percent of all VD infections (149 out of 470), and in the following year had fallen to 25.5 percent (118 out of 463). By 1910/11, though, the number of syphilis cases had exceeded the gonorrheal by 170 patients. It now accounted for 57 percent of all STD patients (399 out of 700), while gonorrhea accounted for 32.7 percent (229 out of 700; see appendix, table 7).

Similarly, syphilis became the most common form of VD for whites near the end of colonial rule. In 1908/09, 38 percent (97 out of 256) of all venereal patients suffered from syphilis, 31 percent (80 out of 256) from gonorrhea. The following year gonorrhea passed syphilis as the more frequent VD, accounting for 52 percent (174 out of 336) of all STD cases, while syphilis amounted to 38 percent (129 out of 336) of all VD patients (the same percentage as the previous year, but a larger number of syphilitic patients). By 1910/11, the numbers were almost exactly reversed: 52 percent (201 out of 384) for syphilis and 36 percent (137 out of 384) for gonorrhea. Thus, while the number of gonorrheal cases had fallen and the syphilitic had risen, the total number of VD patients had grown to 384 (see appendix, table 7).

As in the other African colonies, gonorrhea and syphilis were the two most prominent venereal diseases in German East Africa. Among Europeans, gonorrhea was the more prevalent, except in 1903/04. In that year, there were 28 cases of syphilis to 3 of gonorrhea; there were also more patients with ulcus molle (12) than gonorrhea. However, in subsequent years, gonorrhea was more widespread, rising to 145 cases in 1910/11 before dropping slightly to 136 in 1911/12. Incidents of syphilis also increased over time, from 26 in 1904/05 to 80 in 1911/12. Looking at the entire colony, ulcus molle and bubo were also fairly common among European patients (see appendix, table 10).

Similar to the European population, gonorrhea and syphilis constituted the two largest types of venereal infections for "coloreds." Cases of ulcus molle and epididymitis also had high numbers by the end of the colonial period, but significantly lower than gonorrhea and syphilis. For example, in 1903/04, there were 495 reported cases of gonorrhea and 235 of syphilis, while 180 were recorded for ulcus molle and 53 for epididymitis. Over time, syphilis passed gonorrhea as the most common type of VD among non-Europeans. Indeed, by 1911/12, there were 1,016 gonorrheal patients and 1,220 syphilitic, or 46 percent of all venereal infections (2,650). Gonorrhea in that year accounted for 38 percent. In that same year, only 8 percent of all VD patients were infected with ulcus molle (213) and 5.6 percent with epididymitis (146; see appendix, table 10).

Meanwhile in the Pacific, statistical evidence, even though it was at times irregular and inconsistent as in Africa, nonetheless indicated that VD was widespread and for the most part on the rise. This was particularly true in the territories of German New Guinea, which was comprised of the Old Protectorate (Kaiser-Wilhelmsland, New Pomerania, and New Mecklenburg) and the Island Territories (the West and East Caroline, Marshall, Mariana, and Palau Islands). One medical official stated that venereal diseases had become a "plague" in the colony.[31] Records from the Old Protectorate revealed that the number of VD cases among both "Europeans" and "coloreds" had increased from 1903/04 to 1911/12, though among whites the numbers were not necessarily high. Nonetheless, the numbers rose and VD did appear to spread throughout the colony. In 1903/04, physicians reported 13 "European" cases of venereal disease in Herbertshöhe (present-day Kokopo) and Friedrichs-Wilhelmshafen (today Madang). By 1911/12, the number had risen to 43 (or 3.3 times) and included all the districts in the Old Protectorate (see appendix, tables 13–14). During roughly the same period, the adult European population in the entire colony (both the Old Protectorate and the Island Territories) had grown from 645 (547 men, 102 women) in 1904 to 1,158 (893 men, 265 women) in 1912,[32] or by 1.8 times. Thus, while there were not necessarily numerous VD cases among Europeans, they increased at a higher rate than the population growth.

In Herbertshöhe, the capital until 1910, the number of Europeans infected with venereal disease rose until Rabaul became the administrative center for the colony. In 1903/04 Herbertshöhe, there were 9 VD infections among approximately 320 whites (or nearly 3 percent of the population). By 1908/09, shortly before the capital moved, doctors treated 15 individuals out of an adult population of 386 (or 3.9 percent). The following year only 7 cases were reported, while the numbers rose in Rabaul over the subsequent years. In 1909/10, there were only 10 reported cases. By 1911/12, the figure had increased to 18 among an adult population of 385 (277 men, 108 women),[33] or 4.7 percent (see appendix, table 14).

When compared to other contagious illnesses, venereal diseases had one of the higher morbidity rates in the Old Protectorate. For example, in the last reporting year, VD, with 44 cases, was a distant second behind malaria, which had 130 patients in 1911/12. Nevertheless, venereal diseases accounted for 6 percent of all registered cases. This was slightly more than two years earlier, when 5.6 percent of Europeans reported suffered from VD. As a group in 1909/10, venereal infections (17 cases) were third among the infectious diseases after malaria (88) and dysentery (19). In 1903/04, venereal diseases only accounted for 1.4 percent of all reported patients. That year there were only 13 cases, far behind malaria, which had 213.[34]

In the Island Territories, where doctors submitted data intermittently, it nonetheless appeared that cases of VD were becoming more frequent, or at least physicians were becoming more aware of their presence as German colonial control expanded across its Pacific islands. In 1903/04, two cases of ulcus molle were reported among the European population in the West Caroline Islands on Yap. By 1911/12, doctors reported cases of infected Europeans on all the Island Territories, with a total of 42 patients. Moreover, the diseases had expanded to include not only ulcus molle, but also gonorrhea, syphilis, epididymitis, and bubo (see appendix, tables 13 and 15). Compared to other contagious diseases that year, VD had the most registered patients (42) among Europeans. The next largest group was dengue fever (25) and then malaria (10).[35]

In Germany's other Pacific possessions, namely Samoa and the Kiautschou Bay concession territory, there were signs that venereal diseases were on the rise in the first decade of the twentieth century only to begin to decline near the end of German colonial rule, at least among the white population. In Samoa, VD appeared to have a limited impact on Europeans. In most years, the total numbers remained in the single digits, but they did spike in the 1907/08 report to twenty-six. The previous year, only five cases were reported, and in the following none appeared in the statistical record (see appendix, table 16).

Within the broader context of infectious and parasitic diseases, venereal diseases among Europeans in Samoa also continued to decline in importance over time. In the years leading up to 1907/08, the overall number of afflicted was relatively small. Thus, in 1904/05, VD had the highest numbers of cases, albeit with only three European patients. This was out of a total of 47 white patients, which was 6.4 percent of all registered patients that year. In 1907/08, VD, with 26 patients, was technically second behind the flu (a broad and rather generic category that had 149 cases), but it was still ahead of whooping cough (15) and yaws (13). As a percentage of all cases, the number had dropped to 3.8 percent (26 out of 686). By 1911/12, the percentage had dropped to 2.6 percent (not only had the incidents of VD dropped significantly compared to 1907/08, but so had the total number of patients, to 151). Further, venereal diseases now occupied third place behind the so-called six-day fever (13 patients) and dysentery (9).[36]

In Qingdao, venereal infections were widespread and especially problematic for military authorities. Initially, the VD morbidity rate among military personnel continued to grow in the territory, passing the rate of the entire German Navy in 1899/1900. The following year, the rate in the territory was 2.5 times that of all naval personnel. After 1900/01 the rate began to fall and by 1904/05 essentially equaled the rate of the navy. However, in the last years of German control, physicians complained about an increase in new VD cases, primarily gonorrhea and syphilis.[37]

Among the indigenous population and prostitutes in Qingdao, venereal diseases were also apparently prolific. According to records from the hospital in Tapautau (the Chinese district in Qingdao), which had beds for ill prostitutes, the VD infection rate in 1903/04 among new patients was 5.5 percent (78 out of 1,424). Overall, European female prostitutes had the highest rate of new cases with 5.8 percent (15 out of 256), while Chinese women had the lowest with 5.3 percent (28 out of 522). Within the new cases among Japanese women (or 35 out of 646), 5.4 percent were diagnosed with a venereal disease. For both existing and new patients in 1903/04, the percentage of VD cases was lower, namely 3.0 percent (104 out of 3,539). Chinese women had the highest: 3.7 percent (45 out of 1,205); European women the second highest: 2.9 percent (18 out of 614, or 2.9 percent); and Japanese women the lowest: 2.4 percent (41 out of 1,710). After the colonial administration opened the hospital for prostitutes in 1906, only ten women on average visited each year, even though it could accommodate sixty patients.[38]

In Shandong Province, which surrounded the concession territory and where soldiers also visited prostitutes, venereal diseases were prevalent. Dr. Kautzsch, a German physician working in the Chinese hospital in Jinanfu (today Jinan), the provincial capital, reported in 1912 that out of 85,670 registered patients 12,585 were diagnosed with a venereal disease (or 14.7 percent), which was second behind skin diseases. The majority of these VD patients suffered from syphilis.[39]

Meanwhile in German New Guinea, there was a fairly consistent rise in the total number of indigenous venereal patients. In 1903/04, there were 67 cases reported in Herbertshöhe and Friedrich-Wilhelmshafen; in 1911/12, there were 362, or an increase of 5.4 times, with cases coming from all the major districts in the Old Protectorate (see appendix, table 13). Similar to the situation with Europeans, the figures rose in Herbertshöhe while it was the capital and then declined around the time the capital moved to Rabaul. Then the new administrative center's number began to increase. For example, in 1903/04, the government doctor reported 53 cases. The greatest number of VD patients was in 1905/06 (71), and then slowly started to fall, dropping considerably between 1908/09 and 1909/10, from 36 to 16. Meanwhile in Rabaul, the local doctor recorded only 38 patients infected with a venereal disease in 1908/09, but the number jumped significantly to 139 the following year. In 1910/11, VD cases rose to 180, then decreased slightly to 152 in 1911/12 (see appendix, tables 13–14).

When compared to other infectious diseases, VD occupied a prominent albeit ambiguous position in the Old Protectorate. For instance, in 1903/04, venereal infections were a distant second behind malaria with only about a quarter of the number of patients: 67 with VD, 287 with malaria. Moreover, out of all patients recorded, 4 percent were infected with VD. However, in terms of average treatment days, venereal diseases ranked highest with 44.6, while malaria only had 5.7 (287 patients and 1,648 days). That year, though, yaws (*Frambösie*) was a close second with 44 days (2 patients treated over 88 days). By 1909/10, VD was still second behind malaria (270 patients), but their numbers had nonetheless grown significantly compared to the rise in malaria cases. More noteworthy was the increase of VD as a percentage of all registered patients, which now stood at 13.3 percent. In terms of average treatment days, the number had dropped to 35.9, but still remained far ahead of malaria, which averaged 9 days (3,337 total treatment days). Dysentery was second behind VD with an average of 24 days (162 patients and 3,888 days).[40] Two years later in 1911/12, cases of venereal diseases had passed the total for malaria (307), but remained second behind mumps (623 patients). Apparently there was an outbreak that year. As a percentage of all cases recorded, VD had dropped to 9.6 percent,[41] which was still noteworthy.

In the Island Territories, one of the first reports of VD among non-Europeans came from the Marshall Islands in 1897/98. In that year, the government physician, Dr. Bartels, noted that there were 175 cases of syphilis, or 25 percent of all patients, and 24 with gonorrhea. Over the years, the numbers fluctuated, primarily as a result of inconsistent reporting from all stations. But by 1911/12, the last published reporting year, the number of non-Europeans infected with VD had reached its zenith with 357 cases with reports coming from Yap in the Western Caroline Islands, Ponape (present-day Pohnpei) in the Eastern Caroline Islands, Jaluit in the Marshall Islands, and Angaur in the Palau Islands (see appendix, tables 13 and 15). Compared to other illnesses, venereal diseases in the Island Territories ranked second behind yaws that year, which had 555 recorded cases. Nearly ten years earlier in 1903/04, the same situation existed with yaws having the most registered patients (63) and VD the second most with 43.[42]

On Samoa, VD among indigenes and the Chinese followed a course similar to the Europeans. Initially, cases of venereal infection increased, only to decline near the end of German colonial rule. In 1903/04, there were six cases for "coloreds" recorded. By 1906/07, the number had risen to 67. Three years later, the most number of VD patients were reported (155). In the following year (1910/11), the number dropped by more than half to 68. The next year, the figure fell to 36 (see appendix, table 16).

Compared to other contagious illnesses among indigenes in Samoa, the decline in the relative significance of VD was even more apparent. In 1903/04, venereal diseases were tied with influenza (6) for the largest number of patients. This meant that 5.8 percent of all recorded Samoan patients suffered from a venereal disease that year (6 out of 103 patients). Two years later in 1905/06, when there were more than three times as many VD patients, the disease was behind dysentery (67) and the flu (57). In addition, the percentage of non-Europeans (both "Polynesians" and "Melanesians," but not Chinese) infected with a venereal disease had dropped to 4.5 percent of all cases (41 out of 915). In 1909/10, when the most number of VD cases was recorded, they were also the largest category (with 8.7 percent of 1,783 reported patients) and even syphilis by itself had the largest number of patients (8 percent). By comparison, there were only 18 cases of influenza, 40 of tuberculosis, and 97 of yaws. In that year, the average number of treatment days for venereal diseases, though, was only 3.5, which was extremely low compared to 1905/06 and 1906/07 (with 15.3 and 16.7 respectively). Nevertheless, it was still one of the highest in comparison to the other contagious illnesses. This was most likely due to the high number of patients classified as "elsewhere" among all the diseases, which was an ambiguous term that could mean patients left treatment before completing it. However, by 1911/12, the 36 VD cases reported by Dr. Glantz accounted for only 4.1 percent of all patients (883), while yaws had climbed to 122 diseased, or 13.8 percent.[43]

Because the Chinese in Samoa occupied an ambiguous position statistically, it was difficult to track the impact of VD. Until 1911, resident Chinese were categorized as "White" in censuses. Nonresident Chinese had their own separate classification. Only in 1911 was a distinct classification created for them.[44] However, in the medical reports, all Chinese apparently had their own section beginning as early as 1903/04 after the "Europeans" and the indigenes. In that year, there were 6 VD cases. By 1907/08, the number had risen to 11. And, over the following two years the numbers continued to rise, reaching 24 in 1909/10, only to drop the next year to 8, and then rise again to 15 in 1911/12 (see appendix, table 16).

In comparison to other diseases, the significance of venereal diseases rose and fell, but overall their impact declined among the Chinese in Samoa. For example, in 1903/04, with 6 cases they had the largest group of patients among the infectious diseases, or 10.9 percent of 55 reported individuals. Several years later in 1907/08, VD ranked a distant third behind flu, which had 217 patients or 24.4 percent of all registered cases (890). Dysentery was second with 19 cases, or 2.1 percent of all patients, while only 18 or 1.2 percent of all patients suffered from venereal diseases. In terms of average treatment days that year, VD was second behind dysentery (which averaged 39.2 days) with 18 days. Influenza patients averaged 10.1 days of treatment. In 1909/10, venereal diseases made up the largest group of contagious diseases with 24 patients (or 4.8 percent of the 505 total cases), second was yaws with 15 (or 3 percent), and then dysentery with 12 (or 2.4 percent). With regards to average days of treatment, VD ranked third with 4.8 days, second was yaws with 5.7, and first was dysentery with 9.5. For all three diseases, over half the patients were declared "elsewhere," which meant that the averages were below normal, especially the venereal diseases, which tended to have a much higher average. By the final published reporting year (1911/12), all the infectious diseases fell significantly in relationship to the total number of patients reported. Among these illnesses, the "6-day fever" had the most patients (18) or 2.3 percent of the 784 cases that year, venereal diseases were second with 15 (or 1.9 percent), yaws had 6 (0.8 percent) and TB had five (0.6 percent).[45]

Similar to the African territories, gonorrhea was prevalent in New Guinea, especially in the Old Protectorate. However, other venereal diseases were common as well. In the case of the Old Protectorate, gonorrhea repeatedly accounted for the largest number of venereal infections among indigenes. Indeed, gonorrhea was consistently the largest group with the exception of 1906/07, when it was second behind ulcus molle. For example, in 1903/04, government physicians recorded 31 cases of gonorrhea among "coloreds," nearly half of the 67 reported for that year. Over the years, the number of gonorrheal cases grew practically every year, passing 100 in 1911/12 with 168 cases recorded, or 46 percent of all VD patients. In addition, ulcus molle was often the second largest type of VD reported, with venereal granulum, bubo, and syphilis also appearing frequently in noticeable numbers in the annual medical reports. After 1908/09, doctors reported numerous cases of genital warts, in particular among the indigenous population of Rabaul. In the last reporting year, epididymitis also appeared as the second largest venereal disease in Rabaul and the Old Protectorate as a whole (see appendix, table 14).

Similar to indigenes, gonorrhea occurred more frequently among Europeans than any other venereal infection.[46] In fact, in most years gonorrhea accounted for the highest number of VD patients. The only exception was in 1904/05 when there were two more cases of syphilis (5) than gonorrhea (3). In addition, over the years the number of gonorrheal cases increased. For example, in 1903/04, there were 7 cases among Europeans, while 24 were reported in 1911/12. Whites were also infected with syphilis and epididymitis, with numbers vacillating between them in terms of which one constituted the next largest group. Further, doctors recorded cases of bubo, ulcus molle, and, extremely rarely, genital warts. None of these diseases ever appeared in great numbers in the medical reports (see appendix, table 14).

Meanwhile, in the Island Territories, syphilis was the most common venereal disease among indigenes. In fact, with the exception of one year (1902/03, when no syphilitic cases were reported), every yearly report demonstrated that over half of all indigenous VD patients were infected with syphilis. In 1897/98, 175 out of 199 patients were diagnosed with syphilis. In 1901/02, 76 out of 145 syphilitic patients were reported. While the following year there were no recorded cases of syphilis, the medical report showed that in 1903/04 there were 41 (out of a total of 43). The 1911/12 medical report included 221 cases of syphilis. After this disease, gonorrhea was the next largest group, but often times a distant second. Most of the syphilitic patients came from the Marshall Islands, though by the final reporting year it was evident that syphilis was present in all of the Island Territories of German New Guinea (see appendix, table 15).

For Europeans, no venereal disease appeared particularly more common than any other in the Island Territories. Occasionally, though, gonorrhea would emerge as the most prevalent. Indeed, in 1908/09, 1909/10, and 1911/12 medical reports revealed that gonorrhea had by far the most VD patients, with the majority of them coming from the Marshall Islands. Occasionally there were reports of ulcus molle, epididymitis, bubo, and syphilis, but when recorded they were relatively few in number. Even in those years and places where syphilis had a high morbidity rate among indigenes, the European population reported very few cases, suggesting that there may have been very little or no transmission of the disease between the two groups (see appendix, table 15).

The venereal infection in Samoa with the highest morbidity rate for non-Europeans was usually syphilis, especially near the end of German colonial rule. In the middle of the first decade of the twentieth century, epididymitis and gonorrhea had high numbers, but after that they dropped while syphilis rose. By 1909/10, physicians recorded 144 cases of syphilis (out of a total of 155 VD patients). In the following years, though, the total number of VD cases fell, syphilis still remained the most predominant venereal disease (see appendix, table 17).

Among the reported incidents of infected Chinese in Samoa, no one disease was prominent. In fact, most of the venereal diseases had less than 10 cases each. One year, though, 10 cases of bubo were reported. Moreover, epididymitis remained consistent around 5 or 6 cases every year and hence one of the more frequent venereal infections. Syphilitic cases were almost always in the minority, though gonorrhea some years competed with epididymitis as the most common form of VD infection (see appendix, table 17).

Meanwhile, no one disease stood out in Samoa among whites. Indeed, in most years cases for the various types of venereal infection remained in the single digits. However, in 1907/08, both gonorrhea and syphilis for whites moved into the double digits. In that year, doctors reported 12 gonorrheal cases and 10 syphilitic (see appendix, table 17).

In assessing colonial public health, doctors collected statistical data from the different territories. Their findings indicated that venereal diseases were, for the most part, spreading and on the rise. This certainly applied to the African colonies and to German New Guinea. In Africa, the notable exceptions were the German colonial soldiers in Cameroon and East Africa. There was also a decline in incidents of VD among military personnel in Qingdao. Among Europeans and non-Europeans in Samoa the number of venereal cases also decreased. Nevertheless, in all places VD was still present and continued to pose a threat to the colonial enterprise.

Doctors, though, did more than collect data to assess the situation. They also created categories both for the different diseases and for the different groups of patients. In doing so, they objectified these populations both medically (as "diseased" individuals) and racially (primarily as either "European" or "colored," and hence as a group). The use of statistical data and ascription of racial attributes (and in some cases class) served to justify the various policies doctors used to combat the threat posed by venereal diseases. In doing so, physicians contributed to defining the colonial order, especially through the assignment of character traits to the different "races."

Notes

1. Asad, "Ethnographic Representation, Statistics, and Modern Power," 82.
2. See for example, Reichskolonialamt, ed., *Die deutschen Schutzgebiete in Afrika und der Südsee 1912/13.*
3. *AkG* (1897): 1.
4. *MB 1909/10* (1911): 191–246.
5. Hüntelmann, *Hygiene im Namen des Staates*, 213.
6. *MB 1909/10* (1911): 224.
7. This estimate is based on the figures from the 1911/12 medical report (which included figures from 1 April 1911 to 31 March 1912) and the 1 January 1913 census report (which put the white population at 1,800). For this latter figure, see Rudin, *Germans in the Cameroons*, 116. The population may in fact have been less, which would mean that the percentage was even higher.
8. *MB 1911/12* (1915): 367–373.
9. *MB 1903/04* (1905): 150–151, 159, 164–165; *MB 1909/10* (1911): 381–384.
10. *MB 1905/06* (1907): 356.
11. *MB 1903/04* (1905): 112–116; *MB 1911/12* (1915): 234–241.
12. The medical report provided no population statistic at the end of the reporting year (March 1912), but according to the 1912/13 annual report, the population in German East Africa on 1 January 1912 (the middle of the reporting year) was 4,866; Reichskolonialamt, ed., *Die deutschen Schutzgebiete in Afrika und der Südsee 1912/13*, 9.
13. In the 1907/08 report, it was noted that "the places, for which government physician were provided, were often not occupied, so that regular reporting was impossible." *MB 1907/08* (1909): 306.
14. Medical Officer, DSWA, Denkschrift zur Bekämpfung der Geschlechtskrankheiten, 5 November 1908, 15–16.
15. *AkG* (1904): 596.
16. *MB 1908/09* (1910): 343, 345, 347; *MB 1910/11* (1913): 601, 604, 608.
17. *MB 1907/08* (1909): 309–322; *MB 1910/11* (1913): 601–608.
18. *MB 1909/10* (1911): 447, 449, 457, 458; *MB 1911/12* (1915): 456–471.
19. Richter, Krankenbreicht, Windhoek, 1 November 1893, 16–18.

20. *MB 1906/07* (1908): 171.
21. *MB 1907/08* (1909): 311, 313.
22. *MB 1905/06* (1907): 389.
23. *MB 1911/12* (1915): 647.
24. The Askari were the black members of the German colonial army in East Africa. They were recruited primarily from southern Egypt, with the first contingent coming to the territory in 1889 as part of the Wissmann Troop, which later became the Imperial Protection Troop. Stefanie Michels, "Soldatische Frauenwelten," in *Frauen in den deutschen Kolonien*, ed. Marianne Bechhaus-Gerst and Mechthild Leutner (Berlin: Ch. Links, 2009), 123.
25. *MB 1903/04* (1905): 117–123; *MB 1911/12* (1915): 234–241.
26. Schnee to RKA, 14 June 1913, BArch R1001/5671, 182.
27. *MB 1905/06* (1907): 203–206; *MB 1911/12* (1915): 456–461, 462–466.
28. *MB 1911/12* (1915): 367–373; *MB 1909/10* (1911): 385–390.
29. *AkG* (1904): 596; *MB 1907/08* (1909): 320, 322; *MB 1908/09* (1910): 350, 351. 348; *MB 1910/11* (1913): 604, 608, 601.
30. *MB 1910/11* (1913): 601–608.
31. *MB 1905/06* (1907): 293.
32. These are figures for the entire colony, including the Island Territories. Reichskolonialamt, ed., *Die deutschen Schutzgebiete in Afrika und der Südsee 1912/13*, 9.
33. *MB 1903/04* (1905): 199; *MB 1908/09* (1910): 357; *MB 1911/12* (1915): 504.
34. *MB 1911/12* (1915): 525–532; *MB 1909/10* (1911): 507–510, 514–516, 523; *MB 1903/04* (1905): 199–201, 230–231.
35. *MB 1910/11* (1913): 577–581, 590–594, 599–603, 605–608.
36. *MB 1904/05* (1907): 263–265; *MB 1907/08* (1909): 504–507; *MB 1911/12* (1915): 614–619. The "6-day fever" was a perfect example of the limits of western medical knowledge. This was the only time it appeared in the annual medical report for Samoa and most likely referred to an illness that physicians could not otherwise diagnose except that it had a fever which lasted six days.
37. Hans Podestà, "Entwicklung und Gestaltung der gesundheitlichen Verhältnisse bei den Besatzungstruppen des Kiautschou-Gebiets," *Deutsche Militärärtzliche Zeitschrift* 38, no. 14 (1909): 580–581; Bericht über den Gesundheitszustand, 1 July 1913, BArch-MA, RM3/6766, 152–153; Wend, Hygienische Massnahmen, 1 January 1913, BArch-MA RM3/6767, 75. There is no surviving statistical data for the white civilian population in Qingdao. See also Eckart, *Medizin und Kolonialismus*, 479; Biener, *Das deutsche Pachtgebiet*, 283.
38. Biener, *Das deutsche Pachtgebiet*, 281; Eckart, *Medizin und Kolonialismus*, 480.
39. Kautzsch, Tätigkeitsberichte für Januar–Dezember 1912, February 1912–January 1913, BArch-MA, RM3/7011, 30, 33, 35–37, 39, 41–42, 44–46, 48–49, 51–52, 54–55, 57, 59, 61–62; Huang, *Qingdao*, 231.
40. *MB 1903/04* (1905): 204–205, 256–257; *MB 1909/10* (1911): 511–513, 517–523.
41. *MB 1911/12* (1915): 525–532. Because the report did not contain the number of treatment days for each individual disease, but rather only the total for all registered patients, an analysis of average treatment days is impossible for this year.
42. *AkG* (1899): 364; *MB 1910/11* (1913): 577–581, 590–594, 599–603, 605–608; *MB 1903/04* (1905): 275.
43. *MB 1903/04* (1905): 299; *MB 1905/06* (1907): 326–329; *MB 1909/10* (1911): 588–591; *MB 1911/12* (1915): 614–619.
44. Wareham, *Race and Realpolitik*, 177.
45. *MB 1903/04* (1905): 299; *MB 1907/08* (1909): 511–514; *MB 1909/10* (1911): 592–595; *MB 1911/12* (1915): 614–619.
46. Davies, *Public Health and Colonialism*, 67.

Chapter 6

Racial Categories, Venereal Disease, and the Colonial Order

While medical reports certainly provided a statistical overview of the health (or actually disease) situation in the different territories, they also typologized patients both as "ill" and as a racial category—primarily "European" or "colored," or, in the Pacific, as "Chinese" as well. As other scholars have demonstrated,[1] the apparently simple act of recording and categorizing the non-Europeans contributed toward their integration into German physicians' understanding of the colonial order, and hence into the German colonial hierarchy. Indeed, according to the scholar Talal Asad, "through statistics … Western representations of modern (i.e., Western) society … are offered, adopted, adapted, and employed" in order "to reconstruct the moral and material living conditions of the target populations."[2]

First, when figures appeared in tables, they were medically categorized as "ill" regardless of their place of origin. This meant that Europeans and non-Europeans deviated from the prevailing perception of "health." From the German perspective, this meant that they challenged bourgeois notions of production and reproduction. Moreover, their condition threatened those that were "healthy." As previously mentioned, this medical conceptualization of "illness" was a result of physicians' training and was therefore not unique to Germany's colonies.[3] In responding to the presence of "disease," doctors, like their counterparts in Germany, treated the infected in the overseas territories as "things" or "objects" to be acted upon: first they were diagnosed and then treated in order to eliminate the threat to the public health.

Second, patients were also classified according to racial categories. For the most part, in the statistical tables, registered patients were either classified as

Notes for this section begin on page 86.

"European" (*Europäer*) or "colored" (*Farbige*). In German New Guinea (DNG), the "Japanese" fell into the "European" category.[4] In all reports, "Europeans" always preceded "coloreds." Moreover, although they may have referenced specific groups in their written reports, according to colonial physicians non-Europeans (except the Japanese) were usually categorized as "coloreds" throughout the protectorates by the last years of German colonialism.

Earlier there were some exceptions, though eventually "colored" did emerge as the preferred term. Thus, while previously some reports from Samoa differentiated between some of the various non-Western groups (e.g., Polynesian and Melanesian),[5] by 1905/06 there was, for the most part, no distinction between indigenous populations throughout Germany's colonial empire in Africa and the Pacific.[6] Similarly, in the 1906/07 Togo reports, the physician in Lomé categorized indigenes as "natives," while his colleague in Anecho used the term "colored."[7] That was the only year this occurred. Otherwise, doctors regularly used the term "colored" for non-Europeans.

A more notable exception was the Chinese. When they were included in medical reports in places outside of Kiautschou, namely in Samoa or in German New Guinea, the term "Chinese" was used, not "colored." The term did come after the "coloreds" in the tables, even though the lists only had sections for "ill Europeans and Coloreds."[8] Only by the 1911/12 report for DNG, in the section "total number treated," Chinese patients were placed in the same category as "non-indigenous natives." Even though under "outcome," they were simply listed as "Chinese," the narrative section explained that this included "sick not indigenous coloreds, like Malayans, Tagalongs [from the Philippines], Indians and other South Sea Islanders," because some diseases affected them differently than "the local natives." Nonetheless, the report did refer to the "non-indigenous natives" as "coloreds," though it was unclear whether this name also applied to the Chinese.[9] One could conclude that it did because not only were both groups in the same category, but also because in other reports "Chinese" were included in tables for the "colored workers" hospital.[10]

Thus, there existed a lack of clarity about whom to include, how, and why. This ambiguity provided health officials with the flexibility to include all subject populations to varying degrees in the "colored" category. Such a situation gave doctors a justification for applying a broader and more uniform set of policies based upon their experiences and objectives in Germany. Consequently, more individuals and groups became subject to disciplinary policies aimed at fighting venereal diseases.

This tendency to apply homogeneity to non-European patients also applied to sex. In the tabulated final reports there were no separate listings for males or females, though this was occasionally mentioned in the narrative part. The 1908/09 medical report for Simpsonhafen (Rabaul), however, did include an overview chart about the "individual illnesses of men, women and children of the different resident races," which included the following groups presented in this order: "Melanesian," "Malaysian or Pohnpei people," and "Chinese."[11] It was an exception, though. Hence, in the statistical tables all indigenes were effectively the same regardless of their ethnicity and sex.

This differed from the findings of George Steinmetz. In his illuminating book, he demonstrated how precolonial perceptions of non-European peoples and the socioeconomic background of colonial officials resulted in different "native" policies in Qingdao, Samoa, and Southwest Africa.[12] However, Steinmetz's focus on the socioeconomic and educational background of physicians could explain the essential uniformity that existed in the statistical classifications. Doctors in Germany had essentially the same training and belonged largely to the same social class. Hence, they conceivably approached and viewed the categories and data from similar perspectives.

For instance, like the various governors Steinmetz investigated, doctors were also exposed to precolonial ideas of the "other." As numerous scholars have illustrated, ethnographic studies and travel literature, as well as encounters with non-Europeans in Germany through world fairs, colonial exhibitions, and traveling shows, contributed to a perception of non-Europeans that was different from that of Europeans. Nevertheless, there were also differences among the various non-European peoples.[13] However, as an apparent result of their scientific training, doctors attempted to bring order to the colonial setting that included all overseas possessions, an order based largely on their bourgeois background. Consequently, colonial physicians adopted a consistent form of categorization that contributed both to the objectification of non-Europeans and to reinforcing the colonial order. Vaughan noted a similar group classification in British East Africa.[14]

As already indicated, in both the statistical and narrative section, "Europeans" always came before those categorized as "coloreds." However, what it meant to be "colored" or even "ill" emerged in large part through the narrative section of doctors' medical reports or in their essays on health (hygiene) in the colonies (in such periodicals as the *Archiv für Schiffs- und Tropenhygiene*). What developed within medical discourse, in particular in the fight against VD, was a fairly uniform picture of the colonial "other." As previously mentioned, there were occasional references to different ethnic groups in the reports. Nevertheless, non-Europeans were most often referred to as "coloreds," and no apparent difference existed in their behavior or in their treatment for VD. The traits attributed to them often coincided with those ascribed to those whites not only in Germany, but also in the colonies that did not conform to middle-class notions of health and respectability, therefore, like indigenes, contributing to the spread of venereal diseases.

In the context of the campaign against venereal diseases, such descriptions appeared most often when physicians tried to explain the introduction and spread of VD. Doctors repeatedly contended in their reports that European culture played an important role in their introduction into the territories. Dr. Mense wrote in 1900 that "the carriers of culture [i.e., European males] bring next to the contributions of civilization … also syphilis and venereal diseases."[15] Two years later his colleague, B. Scheube, at the 73rd Assembly of German Natural Scientists and Physicians in Hamburg, remarked it was undeniable that "the carriers of culture brought along with the blessings of civilization also the curse of syphilis to the newly opened territories. Everywhere it comes on the heels of the explorers, conquerors, sailors and merchants, and moved in with them to those places which until then were untouched by the culture as well as syphilis."[16]

Indeed, numerous physicians noted over the years that VD was either introduced or spread with the onset of German colonialism. For example, Dr. Kersten wrote that gonorrhea in German New Guinea "had already begun its victory march as an inseparable companion of the increasing traffic and invading culture." As a matter of fact, it spread to other parts of the colony from the "centers of culture," namely Rabaul and Herbertshöhe.[17] In Togo, the local German doctor reported that "among the natives stand the Christian civilized, better natives at the forefront of the vencreal infected.... A black clerk in Lomé without acute or chronic gonorrhea is a rare bird."[18]

Therefore, as Europeans increasingly came into contact with indigenous populations, venereal diseases were introduced or spread throughout a region. For instance, one physician on Yap attributed the spread of gonorrhea and epididymitis there to the "exceptionally strong ship traffic" in the region.[19] A similar situation was reported in East Africa, where Dr. Gärtner wrote in the late 1890s that "venereal diseases occur here frequently, particularly in Dar es Salaam and Tanga, where through the bustling maritime traffic the spread of these diseases is achieved. Many are also brought in through Zanzibar."[20]

In other reports, physicians stated explicitly that relationships between Europeans and indigenes accounted for the rise in VD. For instance, in Friedrich-Wilhelmshafen, the local doctor wrote that the high incidence of venereal diseases there was a result of indigenes having "intimate relationships" with Europeans, regardless of whether they were "long or short term."[21] Dr. Schelle in German Southwest Africa stated that "there was no doubt that these venereal diseased [i.e., German colonial soldiers] were contributing to the spread of venereal disease among the native women."[22]

In other parts of the overseas empire, doctors documented that as German control was extended, so did the prevalence of VD. This was particularly notable in German East Africa, where medical doctors in the early 1900s reported the presence of venereal diseases in the various coastal stations and then later in Tabora, places where colonial troops (both German and African) became stationed as administrative authority expanded. The same reports indicated that prostitutes also operated in these places.[23]

According to some colonial physicians, the spread of VD was often the direct result of white male behavior. Dr. Shelle remarked that venereal diseases spread among indigenous women because German soldiers ignored his instructions or did not utilize the prophylactics he handed out.[24] Dr. Hummel attributed this to apathy or indifference among whites. In 1901/02, he wrote that "the absence of a lasting success is certainly due in large part to the apathy of the whites, who very often demonstrate a regrettable indifference toward the risk of infection through sex."[25] Nearly a decade later, his colleague referred to those who did not use prophylactics as the "indolents."[26] Another noted that the "ignorance" of whites also helped spread the disease: "For the whites here the same difficulties exist as in the homeland, most are treated by a private physician, many do not even allow themselves to be treated or at the very least only through a quack (*Kurpfuscher*), or buy medicine uncritically from the pharmacy, or the barber, or the store."[27]

Such behavior was attributed for the most part to the unmarried members of the white working class: "It can and must be openly stated, that foremost among those whites responsible for the spread of venereal diseases are the unmarried men of the working class." In fact, they were accused of contributing more to the spread of the diseases than indigenes. According to the reporting doctor, this was largely due to the fact that most of these men either did not seek treatment or "at best [received] improper treatment from a friend or a quack," which did not heal their illness, but rather spread it more.[28]

One of the primary vehicles for the transmission of VD into other parts of colonial territories was through the expansion of trade routes and the rise in commercial activity that accompanied not only German colonialism, but European colonialism in general. Writing in 1914, Dr. Wick in Herbertshöhe reported:

> The traffic between the different native tribes (*Eingeborenenstämme*) was inhibited and vanishingly small through strife and feuds before the entry of whites. The white man brought peace and in its wake a huge increase in traffic; trade relations were expanded or begun anew, which gave new recovery, new energy to the economic life. But with this traffic smallpox and leprosy, plague and dysentery, syphilis and tuberculosis moved into the same street often unhindered.[29]

A similar experience occurred in Africa. For example, in Cameroon, Dr. Jäger noted that the "colossal carrier traffic" (*Trägerverkehr*) contributed to the dissemination of VD throughout the colony.[30] His colleague in East Africa noted that due to caravans, the population in most places fluctuated, which not only spread the diseases, but also made it difficult to combat them.[31]

Indeed, this movement of people played a pivotal role in spreading VD throughout the territories, including to places previously free of the diseases. One physician in Togo wrote that "women and girls" "bring products from all parts of the southern and middle parts of Togo to Lomé" and then return home with venereal diseases.[32] Often this "increasing traffic," as in East Africa, brought VD even "to the up to now less contaminated regions."[33]

Sometimes specific groups that were part of this traffic, yet had connections outside of Germany's territories, were blamed for spreading venereal diseases. For example, Arab and Muslim populations were specifically pointed out as sources for introducing and disseminating VD in Germany's African colonies. One of the first mentions of this came in 1894/95, when Dr. Gärtner in East Africa wrote that "venereal diseases are numerous in Africa and are brought in by the Arabian culture." He also remarked that "those Sudanese recruited in Egypt also brought many [venereal diseases] with them"[34]—the "Sudanese" to which he referred were the Askaris. Similar criticisms were lodged against the Muslim population in Cameroon, namely the Hausa, an Islamic people closely connected with trade throughout West Africa. In 1905/06, a doctor there complained that "the Hausa contributed to the spread" of syphilis, which was apparently on the rise.[35] Nearly five years later, his colleague in Dume, Cameroon, still blamed the Hausa for disseminating the diseases. "It is well-known, that it is the Hausa who spread venereal diseases throughout the territory."[36]

In the Pacific, responsibility for disseminating the diseases was attributed in part to the Japanese and Chinese. According to Dr. Born, "through the connection with Hong Kong and Japan, the risk of bringing in infectious diseases has risen considerably." He was particularly concerned about "the introduction of venereal diseases, especially syphilis," even more so than the plague and smallpox. He noted that "in this regard Japan is namely very dangerous."[37] In fact, government physicians in Rabaul paid close attention to ensuring that the Japanese prostitutes there did not infect Europeans by requiring them to submit to regular examinations.[38] Meanwhile, Dr. Kronecker had nothing but disparaging remarks for the Chinese and their sexual practices when discussing the medical situation in Qingdao. In fact, he believed sincerely that the world "had a serious duty to protect itself with all its might against an invasion of the Chinese proletariat."[39] In German New Guinea, colonial authorities required Chinese contract workers coming into the colony to undergo medical treatment in a concerted effort to stop the spread of contagious diseases, including VD.[40]

Contract workers were part of the larger phenomenon that accompanied European colonialism, an occurrence that played a role in the dissemination of venereal and other infectious diseases. The recruitment of workers, either from abroad or from other regions in a colony, was deemed necessary to develop some colonies economically due to apparent labor shortages. Indeed, for this precise reason Chinese workers were contracted to work on the plantations in Samoa and the territories of German New Guinea. In Samoa, 3,842 laborers were brought in between 1903 and 1913. A similar situation existed in southwestern German Cameroon, where initially workers were recruited outside of the colony, and then once the administration found ways to use more indigenous labor, the use of foreign workers declined.[41]

Throughout Germany's colonies, doctors saw these migrant workers as a source of venereal infection among the non-European laborers. Moreover, many most likely brought VD home with them after their contract ended, and hence contributed to their spread to other parts of the colonies. In Samoa, German doctors in Apia found cases of gonorrhea and secondary syphilis among the Chinese migrant laborers.[42] In DNG, one physician remarked that VD accounted for 8.7 percent of all diseases among "coloreds," most of whom were "workers from different firms." He also noted that a significant number of the new cases came from the "newly acquired workers" (*neue Angeworbenenen*).[43]

Governor Hahl in DNG was also concerned about the impact migratory labor was having on the reproductive capacity of indigenous women in New Mecklenburg. "As the only part of the Old Protectorate where women could be persuaded to sign indentures, New [Mecklenburg] was the colonists' principal source of cheap female laborers, household servants and concubines." Between 1905 and 1907, 475 women left New Mecklenburg to work in the northeastern part of New Pomerania and around Kaiser-Wilhelmshafen. An additional 150 worked "elsewhere in the colony and in Samoa." Reports indicated that these women "brought venereal diseases back" home "after service with the whites," a situation that some colonial officials believed contributed to the decline of the indigenous population on New Mecklenburg.[44]

Blaming non-Europeans for the spread of venereal diseases, even though it was often the result of European imperialism, was part of the larger phenomenon of placing most of the responsibility for their introduction and dissemination on the character traits of these non-European populations. Indeed, Ludwig Külz noted that syphilis along with alcoholism and tuberculosis, diseases associated with German urban centers and the working classes, were "unambiguously racial diseases" (*Rassenkrankheiten*) in the colonial setting.[45] His colleagues used various terms, at times apparently interchangeably, to describe indigenes, such as possessing "loose morals" and being "indifferent," "ignorant," "superstitious," "unhygienic," and/or "indolent"—all of which contributed to objectification and would ultimately justify the various actions taken to combat VD.

Perhaps the greatest complaint leveled against indigenes was that they lacked morals, leading to a spread of VD: "Civilization is indeed responsible for bringing [them in], but not for their general dissemination. This requires a suitable soil, that is, 'loose morals' … that do not allow for immunity."[46] His colleague, Dr. Becker in German East Africa, noted several years earlier in 1895/96 that "to fight venereal diseases … is extraordinarily difficult due to the lax morals of the colored population."[47]

From the perspective of German physicians, this moral condition led to behavior that contributed to diffusion of the diseases. For instance, Dr. Liebl in Togo attributed the rise in VD to polygamy among the indigenous population.[48] In nearby Cameroon, Dr. Zupitza in 1905/06 remarked that "because the indigenous population everywhere is strongly contaminated, above all with gonorrhea, a … decline in venereal diseases" was not likely to happen due to the "coloreds" "relaxed conception of sexual intercourse."[49]

Physicians expressed similar criticisms of the non-European populations' in the Pacific sexual comportment. For example, in the West Caroline Islands, one doctor saw the "loose family ties" as a cause for the "spread of venereal diseases," which also apparently played a salient role in the decline of the local population.[50] Dr. Born in the Marshall Islands remarked that the "free sexual relations" there resulted in the increase in VD, "especially syphilis."[51] Meanwhile, in Qingdao, Dr. Franz Kronecker described the Chinese, above all the men, as possessing "disgusting sexual excesses," which along with "dirt and vermin" necessitated efforts to separate them from the European population out of fear of spreading diseases.[52]

Doctors often pointed to autochthonous indifference toward venereal infections as being responsible for their spread. In Togo, Dr. Krüger reported in 1909/10 that "venereal diseases are very common" and spread as a result of indigenous "indifference (*Gleichgültigkeit*) towards" them. Due to this "indifference," patients often left before the "end of the treatment" and also resumed "sexual intercourse" before they were cured.[53] Several years earlier, the government physician there provided a similar explanation, blaming the "extraordinary indifference ... of the Africans ... towards these diseases" as the "reason for [so many cases reaching] the chronic stage as well as the many secondary illnesses."[54] A doctor in German East Africa described this "indifference" among indigenes as being directed "towards themselves," which nonetheless had the same outcome, namely not seeking treatment or not staying in it until they were healed.[55]

The same German East African physician noted that the African "ignorance" also contributed to this situation.[56] Indeed, for many German doctors, this condition explained indigenous attitudes toward venereal diseases. For example, a medical official in Cameroon noted that "the ignorance of the colored ill" prevented them finding the "correct healing (*Ausheilung*)" for the disease.[57] Specifically, Dr. Jäger remarked that the Bulu in southern Cameroon believed "that gonorrhea was healed when it no longer caused pain."[58] His colleague in Togo noted a similar situation when he reported the comments made by an "older, respected and otherwise intelligent native," who supposedly stated, "One does not have to treat every case of gonorrhea, because there are two types, a non-dangerous one and a dangerous one."[59] According to a doctor in the Marshall Islands, this ignorance even resulted in indigenous females treating themselves "according to indigenous ways." The outcome of this was that later they were "afflicted with chronic gonorrheal cervical catarrh [inflammation of the mucus membrane] and other catarrhs" and ensured a "thorough proliferation of the suffering."[60]

At times German medical officials explained indigenous "ignorance" by pointing out their apparent "superstitious" beliefs or lack of Western education. For instance, Dr. Jäger in Cameroon wrote that "superstition stands like a wall opposed to the efforts of the doctor to spread enlightenment about the dominant diseases."[61] Meanwhile, military physician Dr. Schelle in DSWA remarked that after a meeting between local leaders and colonial authorities to discuss the spread of VD in the colony, it was apparent that many in both groups did not understand the illnesses. He reported that the views of the "natives" could not be taken "seriously," while those of "educated whites" were distant from the "truth and reality." Nevertheless, he wrote that the latter applied more "to the people (*Volk*), to the mass of uneducated"—i.e., to Africans. For him, the primary reason for this was that their interpretation lacked empirical evidence, i.e., they did not possess the same scientific background as German doctors. Consequently, "the native treated gonorrhea, but naturally like all quacks (*Kurpfuscher*)—including the white ones—only the symptoms." They did not have the knowledge to determine whether the disease was really healed or not.[62] Thus, he equated those practicing "quackery" in Germany with "native" healers in Africa.

Another trait attributed to indigenes that helped explain the spread of VD was their "laziness." In 1904/05, the military physician Dr. Schörnich in East Africa wrote that "from Tabora, Bukubo, Usumbura and Schirati it is reported about the increase in venereal diseases among the indolent natives."[63] A few years later, his successor complained that the "indolence of the natives with regards to these diseases" made it impossible to undertake "an energetic campaign" against them.[64] Meanwhile in Cameroon, Dr. Jaeger reported that the "indolence" of the local population was a major hindrance to educating them about the major diseases, including VD.[65]

In ascribing these different traits to the various non-European populations, colonial doctors used language similar to that utilized to describe those Germans who endangered the health of nation, both in Germany and in the colonies. Both non-Europeans and lower-class whites were seen as "lazy," "indifferent," "ignorant," and lacking in scientific knowledge. They also purportedly possessed lax morals. Thus, neither group conformed to middle-class ideals of education and respectability.[66] Of course, non-Europeans also had other qualities attributed to them, including being superstitious.

Nevertheless, like lower-class whites, doctors created an identity for non-Europeans through their discourses in the narrative sections of medical reports. Consequently, they possessed agency that was capable of challenging the values that upheld German colonial rule. The cornerstones of German society, both at home and in the overseas territories, were bourgeois norms.[67] There was, however, a difference between these two milieus. In the colonial setting, these characteristics were ascribed not to a class "other," but rather to a racial "other." In other words, while in Germany the values associated with a healthy nation had a distinctive class identity, these same standards in the colony had a decidedly racial component that drew upon white, albeit bourgeois, norms. A foundation of German colonial rule, therefore, was based on middle-class values of public health tied to concepts of race. Challenges to the vitality of the colonies were also potential threats to the entire colonial enterprise because they possibly endangered the foundations of white rule.

Doctors' perceptions of indigenes played a salient role in medical discourse, especially when statistical evidence did not support the prevailing perception of them. As in Germany, statistical data in the colonies was incomplete. This was especially true with regards to the size of the indigenous populations in the different territories, which often had to be estimated due to the limited extent of formal German rule in some places or the unwillingness of indigenes to cooperate.[68] Medical reports were also deficient because they only included those individuals who actually sought medical assistance from a reporting physician or hospital. For example, the table compiled in 1906/07 for "ill Europeans and coloreds" in Douala only included those in the local government hospital.[69] Similarly, the 1909/10 table printed for "ill coloreds" in Herbertshöhe only provided figures for those found in the government hospital. In Southwest Africa, Governor Seitz reported to the Imperial Colonial Office in 1912 that some whites and "natives" used private physicians who did not feel obliged to submit reports.[70] In addition, some doctors did not submit reports on a regular basis. For example, for several years during the Herero and Nama Wars no report was published, or only the list of white civilians who had died was provided.[71]

Despite this deficiency, which several physicians acknowledged, colonial doctors would comment on the state of venereal diseases in the colonies based upon their views of non-Europeans. Consequently, because of the traits ascribed to indigenes, VD was often perceived as being more widespread than statistical evidence indicated. For instance, at the beginning of the twentieth century, Dr. Heuermann believed that even though few cases had been reported in Cameroon, "the colony was strongly contaminated (*verseucht*) with gonorrhea and syphilis."[72] Nearly a decade later, the government physician in Anecho, Cameroon, reported, "those in the listed venereal diseases for coloreds have no statistical value, because venereal diseases of all types are extraordinarily widespread here." He continued by stating that indigenous practices, such as polygamy and ignorance played a salient role in their proliferation.[73] In Southwest Africa, Dr. Mayer argued in 1910/11 that "to give statistical documentation of objective meaning is … entirely meaningless." He wrote that "not only is every doctor, but also every observant layperson convinced of the almost prodigious spread of sexually transmitted diseases in our protectorate, primarily among the natives." Indeed, he believed that the cases reported that year "on no account correspond to the true number of existing cases." For him, some of the reasons included indigenous and white behavior as well as the limitations of examining all the African populations.[74]

No segment of the population epitomized more the dual medical and racial objectification than indigenous female prostitutes, at least within the context of the campaign to stop the spread of venereal diseases. As in Germany and in other European colonies as well,[75] VD was closely associated with prostitution. Indeed, German colonial physicians saw prostitution as the main vehicle for the introduction and spread of VD. Dr. Mense wrote in 1900 that "the introduction and dissemination [of venereal diseases] is ascribed to prostitution."[76] When they were registered with a hospital or clinic, they became a medical statistic, an object to be diagnosed and if necessary cured. Like their counterparts in Germany, they lacked agency.

However, prostitutes, as indigenous females, were also objectified as a group, and consequently had traits ascribed to them that ostensibly threatened the public health. In this way, they were differentiated from men, unlike in the statistical tables. From the perspective of German doctors, they were seen as sexually promiscuous. As a matter of fact, in the colonial setting, medical officials essentially viewed all women with an overactive sexuality and therefore all of them were suspected of prostitution. This applied to both unmarried and married women. Admittedly, non-European men were also sexualized. On several occasions colonial doctors noted that imprisonment was often necessary to prevent infected African men from having sexual intercourse with women, but at times this was not even enough.[77] However, as Megan Vaughan has already demonstrated within the context of VD, the sexualized woman occupied the more prominent position in the rhetoric. In British East Africa, she did show that the image of the female changed over the decades, but in Germany's colonies it ostensibly remained constant.[78]

This sexual objectification of women was also reinforced by German descriptions of how indigenous males supposedly treated their women. For example, a doctor in Lomie, Cameroon, noted that "the peculiar social position of women, which without their own free will in all things are dependent on their owners, contributes much to the spread of venereal diseases. The same [the owner] permits anyone he sees fit, with or without pay, to have sexual intercourse with his wife."[79]

In a very real sense, then, these German officials adopted contemporary perspectives of non-European women and applied them in the colonial environment. In Germany, the image of the "Hottentot Venus" was associated with prostitutes because the former's perceived overactive sexuality became a vehicle to describe the assumed sexual behavior of white prostitutes. Moreover, both the "Hottentot Venus" and the prostitute were associated with venereal disease. They were both objects of desire and objects of infection.[80] With the advent of German colonialism and the need to combat the spread of VD, this image of the "Hottentot Venus" was essentially reintroduced into the colonial setting as a means to explain and justify health measures introduced to combat the spread of venereal infection.

In developing a policy to prevent the proliferation of sexually transmitted diseases, colonial physicians pursued a number of strategies that drew upon the medical and racial conceptualization of these patients (which not only coexisted with one another, but often overlapped and interplayed with each other) to combat this danger. Thus, doctors needed to respond to the threat posed by VD to German colonialism, which also included addressing the "inappropriate" behavior practiced by segments of the colonial population, both of whites and non-Europeans. Similar to the situation in Germany, most of their efforts were focused on the body of the prostitute. However, due to the nature of the colonial environment, doctors were able to include a much broader spectrum of the population in their measures. These policies ranged from preventative, educational initiatives to more surveillance and disciplinary actions. The objectification of these individuals and groups justified the implementation of these various measures, which aimed to bring about the subjectification of these targeted groups. The more punitive policies included the regulation of prostitution, requisite health examinations of various segments of the colonial community, forced treatment if found infected, and even confinement if unwilling to complete the cure. While implementing these policies, health officials met with uneven success, for much of it depended on the cooperation of the targeted populations.

Notes

1. Kertzer and Arel, "Censuses, Identity Formation, and the Struggle for Political Power," 3, 5; Levine, *Prostitution, Race and Politics,* 199–200; Sean Hawkins, *Writing and Colonialism in Northern Ghana: The Encounter between the LoDagga and "the World on Paper"* (Toronto: Toronto University Press, 2002), 10. See also Alexandra Widmer, "The Effects of Elusive Knowledge: Census, Health Laws and Inconsistently Modern Subjects in Early Colonial Vanuatu," *Journal of Legal Anthropology* 1, no. 1 (2008): 92–116.
2. Asad, "Ethnographic Representation, Statistics, and Modern Power," 84.
3. For instance, Philippa Levine, *Prostitution, Race and Politics,* 200.
4. *MB 1911/12* (1915): 508.
5. For example, compare *MB 1904/05* (1907): 263–265 and *MB 1905/06* (1907): 326–329.
6. The 1908/09 and 1909/10 medical reports for the "colored workers" hospital in Friedrich-Wilhelmshafen had the categories "Chinese," "Malayan," and "Melanesian." *MB 1908/*09 (1910): 606, 407; MB *1909/10* (1911): 523.
7. *MB 1906/07* (1908): 150, 158.
8. For example, see *MB 1911/12* (1915): 525–532, 614–619.
9. *MB 1911/12* (1915): 509.
10. *MB 1908/09* (1910): 404–407.
11. *MB 1908/09* (1910): 382–383.
12. Steinmetz, *The Devil's Handwriting.*
13. For example, see Fatima El-Tayeb, *Schwarze Deutsche: Der Diskurs um "Rasse" und nationale Identität 1890–1933* (Frankfurt: Campus, 2001); Sadj, *Das Bild des Negro-Afrikaners*; and Gilman, *Difference and Pathology.*
14. Vaughan, *Curing Their Ills,* 11.
15. C. Mense, "Syphilis und venerische Krankheiten in den neu der Kultur erschlossenen Ländern besonders Afrika," *ASTH* 4, no. 2 (1900): 104–105.
16. B. Scheube, "Die venerische Krankheiten in den warmen Ländern (Fortsetzung und Schluss)," *ASTH* 6, no. 7 (1902): 233.
17. Kersten, "Gonorrhöe im Bezirk Rabaul," 180–181.
18. *MB 1906/07* (1908): 138.
19. Sunder, Krankheiten auf Yap, 12 April 1901, BArch R1001/5775, 41.
20. *AkG* (1899): 353. See also Liebert to Foreign Office, Colonial Department, 20 July 1900, BArch R1001/5745, 28.
21. *MB 1903/04* (1905), 227.
22. *MB 1906/07* (1908): 171.
23. *AkG* (1902–1903): 388; *AkG* (1904): 46, 53, 55, 554.
24. *MB 1906/07* (1908): 172.
25. *AkG* (1904): 100.
26. *MB 1911/12* (1915): 655–656.
27. *MB 1910/11* (1913): 586.
28. *MB 1910/11* (1913): 587.
29. Dr. Wick, Arbeiterfürsorge in Deutsch-Neuguinea, 1914, BArch R1001/5773, 36.
30. *MB1911/12* (1915), 420.
31. *MB 1905/06* (1907): 357.
32. Ibid.: 198–199; *MB 1904/05* (1907): 118.
33. *MB 1907/08* (1909), 77.
34. *AkG* (1897): 33.
35. *MB 1905/06* (1907): 182.
36. *MB 1909/10* (1911): 328.
37. *AkG* (1904): 620–621.
38. Davies, *Public Health,* 68; Firth, *New Guinea,* 117.

39. Kronecker, "Fünfzehn Jahre Kiautschou," 11–12.
40. *MB 1911/12* (1915): 502–503; Krümling to Vice-Governor Berg, 19 February 1907, NAA G2/H13, 29–30.
41. Eckart, *Medizin und Imperialismus,* 450–451; Firth, *New Guinea,* 112–113, 116, 125; Mark Delancey, "Health and Disease on the Plantations of Cameroon, 1884–1939," in *Disease in Africa: An Introductory Survey and Case Studies,* ed. David Patterson and Gerald Hartwig (Durham, NC: Duke University Press, 1978), 153–154, 156.
42. Delancey, "Health and Disease," 174; *MB 1903/04* (1905): 300.
43. *MB 1906/07* (1908): 208–209.
44. Firth, *New Guinea,* 125; Dr. Wick, Arbeiterfürsorge in Deutsch-Neuguinea, 1914, BArch R1001/5773, 38; *MB 1908/09* (1910): 418–420.
45. Külz, "Grundzüge," 80.
46. J. H. F. Kohlbrugge, "Syphilis in den Tropen 1900," *ASTH* 4, no. 4 (1900): 219
47. *AkG* (1898): 634.
48. *MB 1908/09* (1910): 282.
49. *MB 1906/07* (1908): 323.
50. *MB 1911/12* (1915): 565, 564.
51. *MB 1909/10* (1911): 539.
52. Kronecker, "Fünfzehn Jahre Kiautschou," 11–12.
53. *MB 1909/10* (1911): 397.
54. *MB 1908/09* (1910): 261.
55. *MB 1904/05* (1907): 46.
56. Ibid.
57. *MB 1905/06* (1907): 157.
58. Jäger, "Beiträge zur Rassenhygiene aus dem Bezirk Ebolowa (Südkamerun)," *ASTH* 16, no. 10 (1910): 334.
59. *MB 08/09* (1910): 282.
60. Ibid., 445.
61. Jäger, "Beiträge zur Rassenhygiene," 335.
62. Schelle, Äusserungen zu Protokoll über die Besprechung des Gouverneurs mit den Vorleuten der Eingeborenen, 23 November 1908, BArch R151F/H.ii.h.i, 54–55.
63. *MB 1905/06* (1907): 359.
64. *MB 1907/08* (1909): 77.
65. Jäger, "Beiträge zur Rassenhygiene," 335.
66. Sauerteig, "Medizin and Moral," 57, 67. For the socioeconomic background of physicians, see Paul Weindling, "Bourgeois values, doctors and the state," 198–223; Huerkamp, *Der Aufstieg der Ärzte,* especially 68–70.
67. This class component in German colonialism in other contexts is explored in Walther, *Creating Germans Abroad*; Walther, "Sex, Race, and Empire, 45–72.
68. Sauerteig, *Krankheit, Sexualität, Gesellschaft,* 68–82; Reichskolonialamt, ed., *Die deutschen Schutzgebiete in Afrika und der Südsee 1912/13,* 37, 41-4346-49, 58; Firth, *New Guinea,* 113.
69. *MB 1906/07* (1908): 101.
70. *MB 1909/10* (1911): 511; Seitz to RKA, 12 March 1912, BArch R1001/6010, 61–62.
71. For example, see *MB 1903/04* (1905) through *MB 1906/07* (1908) under "Deutsch-Südwestafrika."
72. *MB 1905/06* (1907): 389.
73. *MB 1908/09* (1910): 282.
74. *MB 1910/11* (1913): 586–587.
75. Stoler, *Race and the Education of Desire,* 129, 179; Levine, *Prostitution, Race and Politics.*
76. Mense, "Syphilis und venerische Krankheiten," 108. See also Scheube, "Die venerischen Krankheiten in den warmen Ländern (Fortsetzung)," *ASTH* 6, no. 6 (1902): 199.

77. Erdland, *Die Marshall-Insulaner,* 118, 124, 131ff., 197, 266; De Groot, "'Sex' and 'Race,'" 89–128; Gilman, "Black Bodies, White Bodies," 213, 216; Gilman, "Black Sexuality and Modern Consciousness," 39; Tobin, "*Venus von Samoa,*" 192–220, especially 207–209; Sadj, *Das Bild des Negro-Afrikaners,* 144–149; Liste der Frauen in Kamina, die verdaechtig erschienen oeffentliche Maedchen zu sein, zur Untersuchung auf Geschlechtskrankheiten, Togo, 17 February 1914, BArch R150F/FA3/1252: 17; *AkG* (1904): 109; *MB 1905/06* (1907): 364, 391, 404; *MB 1908/09* (1910): 510–511; Firth, *New Guinea,* 117, 126; Mense, "Syphilis und venerische Krankheiten," 108; El-Tayeb, "Verbotene Begegnungen," 90; *MB 1908/09* (1910): 215; *AkG* (1898): 634.
78. Vaughan, *Curing Their Ills,* 19–23, 129–154. The change Vaughan notes takes place after World War I, when Germany had lost its colonial empire. Currently no comprehensive research exists on the perception of non-European female sexuality in Germany's colonies.
79. *MB 1908/09* (1910): 216.
80. Gilman, "Black Bodies, White Bodies," 202–242; Gilman, "Black Sexuality and Modern Consciousness," 39.

PART III

Fighting Venereal Disease in the Colonies

Chapter 7

Preventative Measures

As Megan Vaughan pointed out in her study of colonial Nyasaland, medical discourse "could be used to pathologize the African as a social being, and to represent difference in such a way as would provide a clear rational for domination to those who wished to find it ... [and] to satisfy the liberal conscience ... which represented anything 'medical' as an act of benevolence, and even of salvation."[1] In Germany's territories, physicians cast those who did not conform to middle-class notions of productivity and health as medical and racial "others." This objectification justified doctors' actions to bring about the subjectification of target populations, or at the very least, to reduce the threat posed by venereal diseases to the colonial order. These medical officials believed that because they possessed scientific knowledge, training, and tools, they could educate indigenous societies and lower middle- and lower-class whites in the logic and value of middle-class notions of health and respectability. From the same perspective, they also felt assured in taking whatever steps were necessary to stop the spread of VD. They believed that they knew best. Over time, though, in response to the realities of the colonial situation, these doctors focused more on eliminating the threat to the pillars of German colonialism—namely, to the ruling whites, military personnel, and the non-European labor force.

Like their counterparts in Germany, physicians working directly for the state assumed primary responsibility for public health in the colonies.[2] Thus, similar to their German peers, they pursued measures designed not only at changing targeted groups' comportment, but also at using science to eliminate the diseases. In a 1909 speech held before the German Tropical Medicine Society in Berlin, Professor Claus Schilling[3] stated that "the physician is the most important carrier

Notes for this section begin on page 94.

of modern culture in the colonies … because he represents science in the service of humanity,"[4] a view held by his colleagues in the British and French colonies.[5] He went on to say that beyond this "ideal side of his profession as colonizer," the colonial doctor can also contribute more directly to bringing indigenes closer to Western culture.[6]

His colleague Ludwig Külz stated that the main goal of the physician was to contribute to the continuation of the colonial races. In order "to explore and realize the optimum development conditions for the race" colonial doctors would utilize racial hygiene (*Rassenhygiene*)[7]—a concept that eventually would be radicalized under the Nazis who replaced class with race in Germany as an explanation for behaviors threatening to the prevailing order and committed horrific acts in the name of preserving the race.[8] In the colonial context, Külz argued that promoting racial development was the most important task for racial hygiene,[9] which would rely heavily on "personal and social hygiene" to achieve its goals.[10] An essential component in perpetuating the race was "to raise the health level of the individual and the group."[11] This was essential if the race was to avoid "inferior progeny" (*minderwertige Nachkommenschaft*).[12] However, on no account would the non-European races become the equals of Europeans. "The native shall not and must not become our brother."[13] In fact, Külz maintained that the differences between the races justified German colonial policy.[14]

It was the task of the colonial doctor to promote the health of the indigenous population and the colonies. They argued that "the chief task of colonial hygiene [was] not only to maintain at full capacity the living capital [*lebendige Stammkapital*] of our colonies, but also to utilize ['natives'] profitably through the promotion of [their] physical development and, when possible, to increase [them]." As in Germany with regards to the lower classes, they focused on the productive and reproductive abilities of indigenes.[15] Toward this end they would employ both "social and hygienic" methods.[16] Not only would this include using the latest scientifically based medical knowledge, but also educating the indigenous populations in European values, most specifically middle-class German notions of health and labor.[17]

Thus, similar to their efforts to "civilize" the working classes in Germany, the medical profession in Germany's overseas territories were going to "civilize" the non-Europeans in accordance with bourgeois norms. Toward this end, they would utilize many of the methods employed at home. Consequently, the racial hygienic rhetoric played no significant role[18] except to justify medical control over populations beyond what was possible in the metropole.

Doctors adopted both normative and surveillance methods to combat VD. Both employed disciplinary practices designed to bring about subjective behavior in targeted populations. Toward this end, doctors tried to educate both Europeans and non-Europeans about preventative measures. Meanwhile, surveillance methods aimed to facilitate first the diagnosis of diseases, which could be accomplished by the introduction of regular requisite examinations of targeted groups, and then the compulsory treatment of those found infected. The latter at times required the use of supervised confinement in order to ensure compliance.

Educational efforts targeted both whites and non-European populations and in general had the same objective, which was to replace overall lack of knowledge that prevailed with notions of good public hygiene. For indigenes, doctors desired to supplant non-European, non-scientific concepts of disease and hygiene with Western, scientifically based knowledge. In the case of mainly lower-middle- or lower-class white soldiers, the goal was to inculcate them with the ideals of the educated middle class. From the perspective of health officials, both needed to be "elevated."[19]

Drawing upon their own knowledge and training, physicians would go to indigenous schools and villages, where they and their assistants taught autochthonous peoples about health and hygienic matters,[20] which included information about the dangers of venereal diseases and how to stop their spread. In Southwest Africa, the health office desired to educate "the natives about the great dangers that threaten[ed]" "individuals and the whole tribe through venereal diseases." In addition, indigenes were to learn that they had an important role to play in fighting VD. Toward this end, "doctors, administrative officials, and missionaries" needed to learn "the languages of the natives, because then they can place themselves in their [the Africans'] thought processes and awake in them awareness for our hygienic efforts." Their oral presentations would be followed by the dissemination of information leaflets in the indigenous languages.[21] Similarly, Dr. Born in the Marshall Islands wanted to gain enough command of the local language so that "through lectures and informational leaflets" he could bring about change through education (*Aufklärung*).[22]

Physicians provided colonial soldiers, both white and non-European, with similar information. For VD, this meant instruction about the dangers of unprotected sex, the proper use of prophylaxes, and the importance of regular medical examinations.[23] In Germany, health educators often used models of infected organs to help illustrate their point,[24] but there was no evidence to suggest that this approach was used in the colonies.

In order to promote safe sex, prophylactics were usually available in government pharmacies and sometimes in local businesses. In DSWA, soldiers could receive such disinfectants as Viro and Samariter. From 1904 to 1908, soldiers received 2,189 packages of Viro and 9,770 of Samariter as well as 29,250 condoms. If a soldier became infected without using a prophylactic, he was often punished.[25] The implicit goal of this latter disciplinary policy was to effect appropriate comportment the next time the offender engaged in sexual intercourse.

A few colonial physicians believed that only a significant change in indigenous behavior could achieve long-lasting results. This was particularly true in Germany's Pacific island possessions. These doctors believed that the sexual morality of indigenes had to be altered. For instance, Dr. Busse on Yap in the West Caroline Islands stated that in order to stop the spread of VD, "the purpose of the people must therefore be directed to the creation of lasting marriages" away from free sex traffic, where marriage was often only perceived as a game.[26] Meanwhile, on nearby Palau, the *mongol* system was abolished in 1905 by the local district officer, Wilhelm Winkler, who had medical training. In this system, young women lived in club houses with men, providing them with moral upkeep and sexual services. In return, these women acquired esteem and increased their family's status. However, from the perspective of local colonial and medical officials, this system was a source of venereal infection.[27] After its abolishment, Dr. Born noted that "marriages were concluded again, [and] also numerous older women became pregnant. Today more of a family life begins to develop"[28]—i.e., more stable relationships that reduced the spread of VD and bore offspring. Both of these countered the perceived decline in population.

Most measures, though, ultimately assumed a disciplinary approach that necessitated more physically invasive and simultaneously punitive practices. This meant that physicians needed to determine through surveillance policies who was diseased and who was not. They would then treat the afflicted while also removing them from the healthy population in order to reduce the threat of spreading the infection. Consequently, considerable time and energy went into regularly examining the targeted groups, either because they constituted a significant source of infection or they played a vital role in the colonial order—or in some instances both. The objectification of suspect populations helped justify the punitive measures. The goal of these disciplinary actions, like the educational endeavors, was to bring about a normalization of these individuals and groups. However, the increasing reliance on disciplinary action indicated the limitations of their ability to subjectify them.

Notes

1. Megan Vaughan, "Health and hegemony: Representation of disease and the creation of the colonial subject in Nyasaland," in *Contesting Colonial Hegemony: State and Society in Africa and India,* ed. Dagmar Engels and Shula Marks (London: British Academic Press, 1994), 173–174.
2. Kohlstock, "Ueber die Dienstverhältnisse der in den deutschen Schutzgebieten beamteten Aerzte," *Deutsche Medizinische Wochenschrift* 25 (1899): 33–35; H. Werner, "Die Organisation des Sanitätsdienstes in den ehemaligen deutschen Schutzgebieten vor und nach dem Weltkriege," *Deutsche Medizinische Wochenschrift* 64 (1938): 268–271, 309–313; Emil Steudel, "Der ärztliche Dienst in den deutschen Schutzgebieten," *Beihefte zum ASTH* 13 (1909): 17–31; Claus Schilling, "Über den ärztlchen Dienst in den deutschen Schutzgebieten," *Beihefte zum ASTH* 13 (1909): 33–45; Hans Ziemann, "Über die Errichtung von Tropeninstituten und die Gestaltung des ärzlichen Dienstes in den deutschen Schutzgebieten," *Beihefte zum ASTH* 13 (1909): 46–54.
3. Schilling practiced medicine and conducted research in German East Africa before becoming in 1905 the first director of the tropical medicine division in the Robert Koch Institute.

During World War II he conducted malaria research on humans at the Dachau concentration camp outside Munich. He believed that the pursuit of science was more important than the well-being of his patients. Because of his methods, he was sentenced to death at the Dachau Trials after the war. Marion Hulverscheidt, "German Malariology Experiments with Humans, Supported by the DFG until 1945," in *Man, Medicine, and the State: The Human Body as an Object of Government Sponsored Medical Research in the 20th Century,* ed. Wolfgang Eckart (Stuttgart: Franz Steiner Verlag, 2006), 225–229; and Vivien Spitz, *Doctors from Hell: The Horrific Account of Nazi Experiments on Humans* (Boulder, CO: Sentient Publications, 2005), 105–114.

4. Schilling, "Über den ärztlichen Dienst," 32.
5. Neill, "Transnationalism"; Levine, *Prostitution, Race and Politics,* 61–64.
6. Schilling, "Über den ärztlichen Dienst," 32.
7. Külz, "Grundzüge," 79.
8. The literature on racial hygiene and the Nazis is extensive, but one of the more notable examples is Burleigh and Wippermann's *The Racial State.* Pascal Grosse, in his *Kolonialismus, Eugenik und bügerliche Gesellschaft,* makes more explicit the connection between colonialism, racial hygiene, and National Socialism.
9. Külz, "Grundzüge," 79.
10. Ibid., 80.
11. Ibid., 12.
12. Ibid., 80–81.
13. Ziemann, "Wie erobert man Afrika," 27.
14. Külz, *Blätter und Briefe eines Arztes,* 76.
15. For example, see Medical Official, DSWA, Denkschrift zur Bekämpfung der Geschlechtskrankheiten, 5 November 1908, 15–16.
16. Ziemann, "Wie erobert man Afrika," 4–29, specifically 4.
17. Külz, *Blätter und Briefe eines Arztes,* 20–26, 74, 75. See also Eckart, *Medizin und Kolonialimperialismus,* 57–72.
18. Pascal Grosse comes to a similar conclusion, though without demonstrating what colonial physicians actually did. Grosse, *Kolonialismus, Eugenik und bürgerliche Gesellschaft,* 134–135.
19. Robert Debusmann, "Krankheit im kolonialen Alltag: Ärztliche Erfahrungen und Patientenverhalten in Kamerun, 1890–1930," in *Afrika und die Globalisierung,* ed. Hans Peter Hahn and Gerd Spittler (Münster: Lit, 1999), 223; Neill, "Transnationalism," 327–328.
20. Debusmann, "Krankheit im kolonialen Alltag," 223.
21. Medical Office, DSWA, Denkschrift zur Bekämpfung der Geschlechtskrankheiten, 5 November 1908, 19–20.
22. *MB 1910/11* (1913): 719.
23. *MB 1906/07* (1908): 171; *MB 1911/12* (1915): 564; and Dr. Wend, Bericht ueber den Gesundheitszustand der Matrosenartillerie-Abteilung Kiautschou 1 April–30 June 1911, 1 July 1911, BArch-MA, RM3/6764, 20.
24. For a discussion of the type of education received in Germany during this time, see Sauerteig, *Krankheit, Sexualität, Gesellschaft,* 9–33.
25. *MB 1905/06* (1907): 157; Medical Office, DSWA, Denkschrift zur Bekämpfung der Geschlechtskrankheiten, 5 November 1908, 18–19.
26. *MB 1911/12* (1915): 564.
27. Hiery, "Germans, Pacific Islanders and Sexuality," 304–305; Born, Aerztlicher Bericht über die Palau-Inseln, 1907, BArch R1001/5777, 120–134.
28. Born, Aerztlicher Bericht über die Palau-Inseln, 1907, 120–134.

Chapter 8

Disciplining the Body

Another way health officials tried to discipline the targeted groups was to introduce various surveillance strategies. The goal of these strategies was to bring about the compliance of these groups with practices that promoted the health of the colony. One method included the required examination for those segments of the population that stood under government control, such as military personnel, prostitutes, and non-European laborers. Those found infected were required to undergo mandatory treatment until cured. The surveillance of prostitutes was facilitated by the gradual introduction of a system of registration, the issuance of health cards, and the keeping of records.

As in Germany and the British colonial empire,[1] the primary object of control in Germany's colonies was indeed the body of the prostitute. This was undeniably a result of the prevailing view of prostitution and its association with venereal diseases that existed in both Europe and its overseas empires. Indeed, because of this relationship, doctors considered female prostitutes the main public health threat within the context of the campaign to stop the spread of VD. From the perspective of doctors, the best way to control the spread of VD, therefore, was to control the body of the prostitute. Further, prostitution was the one type of sexual contact that colonial authorities could ostensibly regulate more easily. Thus, while marginalized from society through various surveillance measures, the body of the prostitute was made visible to health authorities.

In Africa and the Pacific, prostitution was broadly defined. In Germany, the connection between female hypersexuality and prostitution was embodied in the "Hottentot Venus" from Southwest Africa.[2] With the acquisition of overseas territories with large indigenous female populations, this perception was exported

Notes for this section begin on page 101.

back to the colonies, especially, but not exclusively, to those in Africa. Consequently, many doctors viewed nearly all non-European women as highly sexualized entities, and hence as prostitutes. Accordingly, in East Africa, the site of the first regular medical examination of prostitutes, they not only included registered prostitutes, but also African wives of Askari. In Cameroon, control was not limited to registered prostitutes, but also to soldiers' wives.[3] In nearby Togo, authorities also carried out a "medical supervision of prostitution,"[4] which also included those suspected of prostitution.[5]

In New Guinea and on the Pacific Islands, physicians regularly examined both prostitutes and female laborers on the plantations (who ostensibly also acted as prostitutes).[6] Dr. Wick, in his memorandum on the care of workers in German New Guinea, noted that "almost all [unmarried indigenes] become infected with venereal disease during their contract period—they are actually nothing other than prostitutes (*puellae publicae*)."[7] These women came primarily from New Mecklenburg (New Ireland) in Melanesia, who according to racial thinking at the time were Negroids. Thus, the perception that these women prostituted themselves was most likely linked to the prevailing views of African women. However, physicians in 1908 Southwest Africa challenged this paradigm. Indeed, in contrast to the statements of others, they argued that married African women generally did "not prostitute themselves." They therefore did not recommend examining married indigenous women,[8] in contrast to their colleagues in West Africa.

In their efforts to combat the spread of VD through prostitution, colonial physicians were aided by the existence of bordellos. Such establishments concentrated sex workers servicing white men in locations that facilitated the medical examinations of the women. In East Africa, for example, officials allowed the construction of the "elongated corrugated iron building" in order to have better control over the health of white men.[9] Prostitutes in DSWA and Cameroon, working in bordellos for whites only, also had to undergo regular screenings. One settler in Southwest Africa actually wanted all African women servicing white clients to be housed in state-run bordellos in order to secure for these men a safe source of sex. Similarly, doctors placed the prostitutes in the Rabaul bordello for nonindigenous male clients under their medical supervision.[10] The bordellos in Qingdao also stood under health control, but the degree differed between the ones for Chinese men and those for whites. The control of Chinese-only bordellos "extended merely to general sanitary measures and laws." However, those establishments that only serviced whites were "subject to strong police supervision," which included a regular examination of the prostitutes.[11]

Regardless of their location, health inspections of prostitutes occurred on a regular basis, usually once a week. For instance, Dr. Wendland in German New Guinea reported that the Japanese prostitutes in Rabaul "were examined weekly at least once by a doctor."[12] In East Africa, most health inspections occurred once a week, at least by 1910. In Dar es Salaam they took place every Sunday. In some places, such as Lindi, doctors conducted them only once a month, at least initially.[13]

After the examination, and if necessary the treatment, physicians recorded the results on a card that prostitutes were required to carry with them at all times. According to Dr. Liebl in Lomé, Togo, "this card already represents for prostitutes quite a coveted and valuable object,"[14] most likely because a clean bill of health was good for business. A similar procedure was followed in East Africa, where health personnel entered the "name of the women, the day, and the result of the examination." It was the responsibility of the chief medical officer to maintain "constant supervision" over this list.[15] In Togo, doctors kept a list of examined prostitutes, which included a note of any venereal infections and the date of their cure.[16] The use of these lists and cards gave physicians a means to discipline prostitutes in good health practices.

In general, the medical examination of prostitutes was facilitated by their required registration with local authorities, similar to the situation in Germany.[17] German East Africa was one of the first territories to introduce such measures. In 1900, Governor Eduard von Liebert issued a decree implementing "morals police control" (*sittenpolizeiliche Kontrolle*) of prostitution in Dar es Salaam and Tanga.[18] A year later, the registration requirement for prostitutes was extended to the remaining places on the coast. Those prostitutes who did not register were to be found and placed under official control.[19] Such regulation could only occur "where the means for an orderly police are available, i.e., in the district offices therefore." [20] In 1910, Governor Freiherr von Rechenberg ordered the "general control of prostitutes" throughout the entire colony.[21] Colonial authorities attempted to introduce similar requirements in the other territories, such as Togo, Cameroon, and Samoa, which were often enforced by police sweeps through some of the larger urban centers.[22]

However, not in all territories did health officials attempt to pursue a systematic effort to register all women practicing prostitution. For example, in Qingdao, those prostitutes who did not work in a bordello were not subject to any medical supervision. Even those that worked in bordellos for Chinese men were only subject to general sanitary rules and regulations. In DSWA, one official in 1910/11 lamented that "not even the black prostitutes are being controlled."[23] Despite this situation, health officials in the colony would occasionally carry out sweeps that would include a health examination of prostitutes. Authorities conducted similar sweeps in other territories as well.[24]

Because military service personnel were integral to maintaining colonial order, military doctors in the overseas territories regularly examined soldiers and sailors—much like their counterparts at home and in the British colonies.[25] The hierarchal nature of the military certainly facilitated the carrying out of health inspections. For instance, naval doctors in Qingdao examined on a monthly basis noncommissioned officers and sailors "for skin and venereal diseases."[26] Similarly, Dr. Gärtner in East Africa reported that "medical inspections take place every month for the troops."[27] In DSWA, where doctors saw white soldiers as a major source of the spread of VD among indigenous women,[28] they examined troops also monthly, but "in order to prevent the concealment of sexual diseases, [the inspections] took place unannounced."[29] Though never explicitly stated, colonial physicians in Cameroon apparently conducted regular health inspections of the German soldiers, as evidenced by the publication of semiannual medical reports.[30]

The examination of service personnel also included non-European soldiers. For instance, Dr. Gärtner in East Africa noted that as early as 1894/95, health inspections for the Askari occurred on a monthly basis, a practice that continued into the next decades.[31] In Cameroon monthly health inspections commenced at the beginning of the twentieth century.[32] However, comments made by the physician in Doume indicated that such examinations were not widespread until later. He said in 1909/10 that "a gradual health inspection of all soldiers ... has to occur."[33] In other parts of the colony, such as in Ebolowa, Kousseri, and Lomie, similar measures were planned.[34] In the 1911/12 report for DNG, Dr. Wendland mentioned that "at all stations an examination of indigenous soldiers ... by the government physician would be carried out,"[35] a practice begun as early as 1902.[36]

In the German colonial setting, medical officials did not limit themselves to prostitutes and military personnel. As a matter of fact, in many of the territories, doctors attempted to expand their medical purview to include those segments of the population connected to colonial control and the economy, especially those deemed to be a source of infection. This was especially the case as VD continued to spread despite physicians' efforts. Because they were dealing with groups that were relegated to subordinate positions in colonial society, doctors could, without legal repercussions and largely with the support of the administration, attempt to exercise control over the bodies of broader segments of the colonial population through required medical screenings.

For instance, doctors in Cameroon saw those associated with trade and plantation work as contributing to the spread of VD. By 1910 they had begun introducing "a systematic control of all" of workers, porters, and traders.[37] In Molundu, on the border with the French Equatorial Africa, the local government doctor also conducted health screenings of newly arrived workers as well as the crew of ships docking on the Dja River.[38]

In German New Guinea, colonial authorities also focused on regulating the bodies of indigenous laborers for venereal diseases. Dr. Wendland reported in 1902 that in the Old Protectorate "workers for the government as well as workers for the New Guinea Company are regularly examined primarily for venereal diseases and scabies," a practice that has been in place for years. Health officials examined male laborers every three months, and females once a month,[39] thus demonstrating the prevailing gender bias. Several years later, doctors examined all Pacific Islander and Asian workers once a month. This included those already working and those newly hired. A similar practice existed in the East Caroline Islands. However, those working for other companies were not required to undergo the mandatory health examinations, though such inspections ostensibly occurred earlier on the plantations around Herbertshöhe. In an effort to reduce the number of VD infections and to prevent its spread, workers were also required to undergo a health examination before returning home.[40]

Such health inspections also included Chinese, whether they were immigrants or contracted workers. Government doctors saw the Chinese as especially threatening and hence examined them medically even before they could land and work. Already in 1902, Dr. Born intended to keep all newly arrived Chinese, and even Japanese, under medical supervision in order to prohibit the introduction of syphilis to the West Caroline Islands. A similar measure was introduced around the same time in Herbertshöhe. Starting in 1903, German physicians in Samoa also screened Chinese contract laborers entering the colony.[41]

The examination of Japanese even extended to the crew of every Japanese ship landing on Yap in the West Caroline Islands. Dr. Born, in his report on climate and health conditions there, wrote that this measure was taken to prevent the spread of syphilis to the island. The health inspection included everyone, "from the captain to the cabin boy."[42] In 1912, the government physician on Jaluit in the Marshall Islands wanted to inspect all crews and passengers for venereal diseases and to forbid the landing of those found infected. However, the colonial administration in Rabaul found such a policy to be in violation of existing ordinances regulating the landing of crews and passengers. From its perspective, such actions on the part of the doctor could have led to "major disagreements" with other countries.[43]

Near the end of German colonial rule in DNG, indigenous prisoners were also added to the list of people whom physicians examined monthly throughout the colony for infectious diseases, especially VD.[44] A comparable situation existed in Togo, where apparently the only males required to submit to health inspections were prisoners, though it did not necessarily apply to the entire colony. In 1911/12, Dr. Simon in Palime noted under the section "social hygiene" that "the prisoners in Palime and Misahöhe were examined monthly for their health."[45] Meanwhile, in East Africa "colored … servants" also had to undergo monthly health examinations.[46]

In DSWA, physicians desired to examine all indigenes, even though Africans were not required to comply. In the 1908 memorandum regarding the fight against sexually transmitted diseases, the imperial government advocated among other policies "a regular examination of all native men."[47] Earlier authorities apparently inspected entire indigenous settlements.[48] By 1906/07, the reporting doctor noted that "in some places a weekly as well as monthly examination of all available natives took place."[49] However, later such inspections became more limited. For instance, in 1910/11, only one in Keetmanshoop was reported that included all the "unmarried [indigenous] men."[50] Colonial health officials recognized that the success of such measures ultimately depended on educating "the natives about the nature of venereal diseases and the necessity of hospital treatment."[51]

Those Africans who worked for private individuals or companies were only sent to the doctor "when something noticeable was detected." After the introduction of self-government in the colony, which included the requirement that local communities pay for services, the situation changed. Now employers sent their workers less frequently because they often had to assume financial responsibility for any medical treatments.[52]

The goal of the examinations was to separate the healthy from the infected so that those identified with a venereal disease could be separated from the fit population until cured. The treatment of VD was facilitated by advancements in medical science, but even these did not always prove sufficient in fighting infections. Moreover, not all targeted individuals complied with prescribed cures. This necessitated more stringent surveillance policies comparable to what officials in the United Kingdom and its colonies were permitted to do, but beyond what German law at home allowed.

Notes

1. Levine, *Prostitution, Race and Politics*; Howell, *Geographies of Regulation*; Stoler, *Race and the Education of Desire,* 129, 179.
2. Gilman, "Black Bodies, White Bodies," 213, 216; Gilman, "Black Sexuality and Modern Consciousness," 39.
3. *AkG* (1902–1903): 388; *MB 1905/06* (1907): 364, 391–392, 404, 438; *MB 1908/09* (1910): 510–511.
4. *MB 1908/09* (1910): 261. See also Polizeimeister, Liste der Kontrollierten für Geschlechtskrankheiten, Lomé, 30 May 1912, BArch R150F/FA3/86, 35; Health Commission, Regelung der Prostitution in Lomé (draft), 1908, BArch R150F/FA3/134, 98–99.
5. Liste der Frauen in Kamina, die verdaechtig erschienen oeffentliche Maedchen zu sein, zur Untersuchung auf Geschlechtskrankheiten, 17 February 1914, BArch R150F/FA3/1252, 17.
6. Firth, *New Guinea,* 117, 126; *AkG* (1904): 109.
7. Wick, Arbieterfürsorge in Deutsch-Neuguinea, 1914, BArch R1001/5773, 38.
8. Medical Officer, Denkschrift zur Bekämpfung der Geschlechtskrankheiten, 5 November 1908, 20–21.
9. Becher, *Dar es Salaam, Tanga und Tabora,* 42.
10. Heim, "Die Syphilis in den deutschen Schutzgebieten," 197; Health Commission, Regelung der Prostitution in Lomé, 1908, 98–99; Oermann, *Mission, Church and State Relations,* 212; *MB 1911/12* (1915): 503.
11. Uthemann and Fürth, "Tsingtau," 25. See also Kronecker, "Fünfzehn Jahre Kiautschou," 16.
12. *MB 1911/12* (1915): 503.
13. *MB 1905/06* (1907): 13, 17, 364; *MB 1906/07* (1908): 13; *MB 1911/12* (1915): 169–174.
14. *MB 07/08* (1909): 251.
15. Imperial Governor, DOA, to all departments on the coast, 8 March 1901, BArch R1001/5745, 56.
16. Liste der auf Geschlechtskrankheiten untersuchten Frauen, Lomé, 26 August 1912, BArch R150F/FA3/94, 30; Liste aufgezeichneten Frauen, die auf Geschlechtskrankheiten untersucht wurden, Atakpame, 16 February 1914, BArch R150F/FA3/1252, 10–12; Liste der vom Regierungsarzt geschlechtskrank gefundenen Frauen, Atakpame, 17 February 1914, BArch R150F/FA3/1252, 36–37.

17. Jenders and Müller, *"Nur die Dummen,"* 30, 36; Sauerteig, *Krankheit, Sexualität, Gesellschaft,* 344. Also Evans, "Prostitution, State and Society," 106–129.
18. Liebert to the Colonial Department, German Foreign Office, 20 July 1900, BArch R1001/5745, 28.
19. Imperial Governor, DOA, to all departments on the coast, 8 March 1901, BArch R1001/5745, 55–56; *AkG* (1902–03): 388; Rechenberg, Governor German East Africa, Verfügung betr. Geschlechtskrankheiten, 1 December 1910, BArch R1001/6040, 136.
20. *MB 1903/04* (1905): 72.
21. *MB 1911/12* (1915): 169; *MB 1910/11* (1913): 178.
22. Polizeimeister, Liste der Kontrollierten für Geschlechtskrankheiten, 30 May 1912, 35; Health Commision, Regelung der Prostitution in Lomé, 1908, 98–99; *MB 1907/08* (1909): 201; *AkG* (1904): 624; Liste der Frauen in Kamina, die verdaechtig erschienen oeffentliche Maedchen zu sein, zur Untersuchung auf Geschlechtskrankheiten, 17 February 1914, 17.
23. *MB 1910/11* (1913): 588.
24. Ibid., 587; *MB 1907/08* (1909): 201; Polizeimeister, Liste der kontrollierten für Geschlechtskrankheiten, 30 May 1912, 35; Health Commission, Regelung der Prostitution in Lomé, 1908, 98–99.
25. Sauerteig, *Krankheit, Sexualität, Gesellschaft,* 344; Howell, *Geographies of Regulation*; Levine, *Prostitution, Race and Politics.*
26. Dr. Wend, Bericht ueber den Gesundheitszustand der Matrosenartillerie-Abteilung Kiautschou 1 April—30 June 1912, 1 July 1912, BArch-MA, RM3/ RM3/6765, 65–66. See also Dr. Wend, Bericht ueber den Gesundheitszustand der Matrosenartillerie-Abteilung Kiautschou 1 January–31 March 1912, 1 April 1912, BArch-MA, RM3/6764, 394–395; Podestà, "Entwicklung und Gestaltung," 576.
27. *AkG* (1897): 34.
28. *MB 1906/07* (1908): 172.
29. Medical Office, DSWA, Denkschrift zur Bekämpfung der Geschlechtskrankheiten, 5 November 1908, 18–19.
30. *AkG* (1904): 73; *MB 1905/06* (1907): 122–123, 389, 391, 404–405, 410, 417, 419, 423, 431, 437, 438; *MB 1906/07* (1908): 314, 320, 323; *MB 1907/08* (1909): 521–522; *MB 1908/09* (1910): 503, 507, 510–511; *MB 1909/10* (1911): 329, 629, 635, 637, 639; *MB 1910/11* (1913): 764–765; *MB 1911/12* (1915): 638, 639.
31. *AkG* (1897): 34; *AkG* (1904): 46.
32. The first discovered mention of these examinations was in a report from 1904/05; *MB 1905/06* (1907): 438.
33. *MB 1909/10* (1911): 328.
34. Ibid., 329.
35. *MB 1911/12* (1915): 503.
36. *AkG* (1904): 109.
37. *MB 1909/10* (1911): 328, 329.
38. Imperial Regierungsarzt, Kurzer sanitärer Bericht über das Vierteljahr vom 1 October–31 December 1911, 24 January 1912, BArch R1001/5763, 161.
39. *AkG* (1904): 109. See also Hahl to RKA, 5 October 1912, BArch R1001/5779, 54.
40. *MB 1904/05* (1907): 165, 218, 238; Viertel-Jahresbericht 1 July–30 September 1910, 10 October 1910, BArch R1001/5772, 25; *MB 1906/07* (1908): 208; *MB 1903/04* (1905): 190. See also MB *1911/12* (1915): 503.
41. *MB 1903/04* (1905): 190–191, 300; Krümling to Berg, 19 February 1907, NAA G2/H13, 29–30; *AkG* (1904): 127.
42. *AkG* (1904): 621.
43. Imperial Government, Rabaul, to Regierungsarzt in Jaluit, 25 April 1912, NAA G2/U24, 12.
44. *MB 1911/12* (1915): 503.
45. Ibid., 447.

46. *MB 1905/06* (1907): 364.
47. Medical Office, DSWA, Denkschrift zur Bekämpfung der Geschlechtskrankheiten, 5 November 1908, 20.
48. *MB 1910/11* (1913): 587.
49. *MB 1906/07* (1908): 172
50. *MB 1910/11* (1913): 587.
51. Medical Office, DSWA, Denkschrift zur Bekämpfung der Geschlechtskrankheiten, 5 November 1908, 19–10.
52. *MB 1910/11* (1913): 586.

Chapter 9

TREATING THE BODY

In the diagnosis and treatment of infected individuals, colonial physicians relied heavily on scientific discoveries. Already by the end of the nineteenth century, they knew the causes of gonorrhea and ulcus molle, and during the first decade of the twentieth century, scientists had found sources for syphilis and other related treponema. In addition, August Wassermann had developed a serological test for syphilis, albeit one that was not completely reliable.

Nevertheless, there were still limitations to their knowledge. For example, doctors at the time were unsure exactly what the so-called six-day fever was. In the realm of VD, they also had limited information about venereal granuloma, a relatively common disease in the Old Protectorate of New Guinea. In a 1903/04 report, one government physician in Friedrich-Wilhelmshafen stated that it was "a contagious disease, as [it] has repeatedly been observed here, where the illness was transferred as a result of sexual intercourse." He was uncertain how much time had elapsed between the initial infection and the manifestation of the disease due to insufficient observations. He nevertheless concluded that "this time appeared to be a longer one."[1]

Like their counterparts at home, with the advance of scientific knowledge, physicians had more information and better tools at their disposal to combat the spread of venereal diseases. In diagnosing patients, colonial physicians used a variety of techniques. Before the advent of serological tests, the primary means of detection was through a physical exam for visible signs of VD.[2] Dr. Born on the Ebon atoll discovered twenty-six men infected with "fresh cases of gonorrhea" "through the general examination." He admitted that it was more difficult to identify infected women because for them the symptoms were "much less mark-

Notes for this section begin on page 111.

edly pronounced." Therefore, he had to conduct a much more invasive examination, but even then the presence of gonorrhea could not easily and accurately be determined. He noted that "because non-gonorrheal diseases of the vagina and the uterus also have a similar appearance such as gonorrhea, and gonorrhea among the diverse bacterial flora in the vaginal secretions in women are much harder to differentiate than in the secretion of the male urethra."[3]

Though not explicitly stated, he most likely used a microscope to examine the women's secretions in order to "eliminate all doubtful cases."[4] Indeed, doctors often used microscopes to determine the veracity of their initial diagnosis. For example, Dr. Jaffé in DSWA, reported in 1907/08 that "in the native hospital primary skin lesions and oozing papules from the majority of those admitted because of syphilis were microscopically examined." Using the latest dyes, "the spirochete pallida are detected almost with every examination."[5]

In 1906, an important diagnostic method for detecting syphilis became available to doctors in Germany. In that year, Wassermann developed a serological test for syphilis, the so-called Wasserman test. The first mention of the test in the colonies came in 1911. Dr. Graf, a military physician in DSWA, noted that "the material for the Wassermann Reaction arrived in the colony in the form of the Dunger modification first in the middle of August 1911."[6] While important as a tool for detecting syphilis in its early stages, the test was not always dependable. It had a tendency to produce false positives for other diseases or someone already treated for the disease or to produce no reaction for an individual infected with syphilis.[7]

Moreover, because they were so closely related, it did not resolve an important medical issue in the colonies, namely the difference between syphilis and yaws. Throughout the colonial period, local doctors often mistook yaws for sexually transmitted syphilis. However, the causes of the two were decidedly different, though the treatment was the same. In some locations, especially the Pacific, this often led to false conclusions about the severity of syphilis. Once doctors became aware that the diseases were caused by different, albeit related bacteria (*Treponema pertenue*), they began to look for different symptoms[8] and even demographic information as a means to differentiate between them. With regard to the latter, Dr. Rodenwaldt in Cameroon remarked in the 1910/11 report that "if all these many cases of tertiary skin, bone, and mucosal diseases belong to syphilis, [and] not to yaws, a significant degeneration of the population would have already occurred."[9]

Some colonial doctors were not satisfied with this technique. One physician complained that the Wasserman test was "too complicated and [did] not work without a large laboratory and animal house." Dr. Born in the Pacific recommended that "as a modern aid to discovering [cases of syphilis] the new Luet intracutaneous reaction should be considered." He noted that its use was "specified by an American doctor" in a recent U.S. medical journal. Born added that "this reaction is supposed to be very useful for the latent stage of syphilis."[10]

This initial uncertainty about the differences between syphilis and yaws, for example, was part of the larger phenomenon of scientists' and doctors' incomplete understanding of diseases. In the early years of German colonialism, for example, physicians did not know whether or not venereal diseases behaved differently in the colonies and in non-European bodies. Once again, then, medical and racial perspectives converged in the effort to determine how different diseases acted in indigenous bodies and tropical climates. In other words, their bodies once again became a site of not only disease, but also of racial "otherness." Repeatedly physicians investigated whether or not venereal diseases were different in tropical environments and whether or not they acted differently in indigenous bodies.[11] The underlying belief apparently was that the diseases might have a different pathology because non-Europeans were racially different.

However, by the end of the first decade of the 1900s, many physicians saw no differences between how diseases behaved and how treatments worked in indigenous bodies and colonial settings. In 1907/08 Cameroon, one physician reported that despite frequent assertions to the contrary, he had much success with "the inunction of mercury among indigenes."[12] However, doctors continued to point out a major difference between non-Europeans and Europeans that contributed to the spread of VD and hence the need to regulate indigenous bodies, namely the prevailing sociocultural conditions in non-European societies. According to contemporaries, autochthonous attitudes, behaviors, beliefs, customs, and hygiene even accounted for the different course of syphilis in the colonies from that in Europe.[13]

Once diagnosed with a venereal disease, the infected were required to undergo mandatory treatment until healed. Out of Dume, Cameroon, one physician reported that "everyone found to be ill is taken into the hospital for treatment and are not released until they are completely healed."[14] This applied to all of those subject to regular health inspections or at times to anyone else found infected with venereal diseases through other means. However, such stipulations pertained primarily to indigenes and white military personnel. In German Southwest Africa, the situation was apparently so bad that Dr. Schelle believed the only way to get the situation under control was to send infected white soldiers home. "Because there was no doubt, that these infected men continued to contribute to the spread of venereal diseases among the native women," the only option remaining for "an improvement in the situation" was "by sending home the infected. Therefore, all those infected with a venereal disease whose expected recovery took longer time than eight week were sent home."[15] Here was another indication of the authority colonial doctors could exercise in contrast to their colleagues at home.

German doctors treated a variety of venereal diseases in the overseas possessions. The diseases diagnosed most regularly included genital warts (*Feigwarzen*), epididymitis (*Hoden- und Nebenhodenentzündung*), ulcus molle (*weicher Schanker* or *Schanker*), bubo (*Bubo*), gonorrhea (*Tripper*), and syphilis (*Syphilis, harter Schanker, Lues*). In the Old Protectorate of German New Guinea, cases of venereal granuloma (*venerisches* Granulum) appeared frequently. Some of these illnesses often described a condition or symptoms and hence revealed that physicians were not always clear what they were and what caused them exactly, such as bubo or even epididymitis. A bubo was common in sexually transmitted diseases and was characterized by "clearly visible and palpable swelling of the lymph nodes, especially in the groin."[16] Epididymitis was an inflammation of the epididymis and was usually triggered by some other venereal bacteria. For instance, Dr. Zupitza in 1904/05 reported that gonorrhea "caused 15 cases of epididymitis" among African soldiers in Cameroon.[17] In another case, syphilis preceded the infection of the testicles.[18]

As in Germany, there was not always a consensus on the best way to treat an illness or at times even what caused a disease. For example, with regard to venereal granuloma in the Pacific, physicians did not know much about it or how to treat it. Government doctor Willy Hoffmann in Friedrich-Wilhelmshafen provided a detailed report in 1903/04 on his efforts to treat the infection in an attempt to share his knowledge with others. He firmly stated that "with syphilis this illness has nothing to do." He concluded, therefore, that mercury treatments were "completely useless."[19]

Consequently, he had to draw upon other knowledge from home in order to find a cure. For him, the "only means to heal this disease" was "to destroy the diseased spot with a knife, scissors, [or] sharp spoon … through cauterization." He also noted with regards to "follow up treatment and the treatment of those non-operated cases [that] besides idoform [a disinfectant] and bismuth etc., … wet bandages with camphor wine, hydrogen peroxide and formalin have proven themselves."[20] The following year he remarked that "the best way to treat venereal granuloma, when possible, is surgically."[21] However, two years later in 1906/07 Dr. Hoffmann apparently changed his approach because he only treated patients with potassium iodide (*Jodkali*) and mercury applications (*Schmierkuren*),[22] medicines commonly associated with the treatment of syphilis at this time. In 1910/11, another government physician used a combination of techniques to cure the illness. First, he used a "sharp spoon" to remove "the diseased inguinal glands," then Paquelin (a form of thermocauterization), which apparently produced good results. He also applied mercury and potassium iodide.[23] The following year, though, Dr. Hoffmann concluded from his experience in Kavieng in northern New Mecklenburg (later New Ireland) that surgery was the most suitable means to cure this disease. Dr. Kröning in nearby Namatanai came to the same conclusion.[24]

For the treatment of gonorrhea, physicians applied the methods used in Europe to treat infected patients in the colonies. For instance, in both locations doctors administered male gonorrheal patients' injections (*Einspriztungen*) or urethral irrigations (*Spülungen*) once or twice a day as part of the cure. This entailed using either a syringe or a bougie to wash out the urethra with such disinfectants or antiseptics as silver salts, including Protargol, or potassium permanganate. Such treatments were usually uncomfortable and even painful.[25]

As in Germany, doctors experimented with other gonorrheal medications and treatments. For example, on several occasions, various types of salicylic acid were tried as an antiseptic, though one physician in East Africa noted that its use was "without success."[26] Another physician in German East Africa, Dr. Lenz, administered internally Santyl[27] in tablet, drop, and capsule form with "good successes."[28] In two particularly severe cases, one doctor in Cameroon ordered that the patients be treated "with opium suppositories, hot hip baths von 38 to 40° [Celsius], later massages and continuous irrigation with potassium permanganate and Protargol," which led to their healing.[29]

For women, a regimen was used that targeted "all potentially infected areas." This meant that treatment was invasive and painful. "The vulva and vagina were thoroughly cleaned, and the ducts of the accessory glands treated with a silver salt, mercurochrome and acriflavine as these became available. Some venereologists irrigated the urethra with potassium permanganate …, while others preferred to instill an antiseptic. Finally, the cervix was cauterized with silver nitrate, or a medicated wick was inserted."[30] Under ideal circumstances, physicians carried out this treatment twice a day. If the infection was more advanced, then additional and even more invasive procedures were required.[31]

For both men and women, but especially for women, the disease was often "left to run its course" (though treatments continued regularly) until tests determined that there were no more gonococci present. This, though, could be difficult to determine in women, and thus many physicians were cautious about females resuming intercourse too quickly. While treatments often led to a complete cure in mild cases, reinfection could always occur, and in more severe instances "remissions and exacerbations" were also possible.[32]

For the treatment of syphilis, colonial doctors also drew upon knowledge and experience gained in Europe. In the later part of the nineteenth century and into the twentieth, physicians in Germany and Europe used mercury and iodide as curative agents. These were also the preferred medicines in the colonies. Indeed, colonial physicians reported repeatedly on the use of mercury through inunction and different formulations of iodine through injections to treat syphilis. Iodine, usually in the form of iodipin, iodoform, or potassium iodide, was utilized as a disinfectant and applied in combination with mercury treatments in more difficult cases or alone either in milder cases or when the use of mercury was deemed inappropriate. In some of the milder cases, doctors sometimes followed up with calomel. However, mercury applications, though often painful and with difficult side effects, were the preferred method for doctors because of their apparent therapeutic efficacy. Scientists and physicians did, though, debate endlessly over how long the treatments should last, what the dosage should be, when to begin the treatments, and how the to administer them. Relapses were not uncommon, and the frequent long treatments were an indication that they were ultimately ineffective.[33]

In 1909, an apparent major breakthrough in the treatment of syphilis occurred when Paul Ehrlich and Sahachiro Hata successfully tested the 606th sample of an arsenical. After releasing it in limited amounts for clinical trials against human syphilis, in 1910 Ehrlich announced publicly that the "magic bullet" (*Zauberkugel*) or "one-shot cure" (*therapia magna sterilisans*) against syphilis had been found with limited side effects. In that same year it was patented under the name Salvarsan and became available on the open market. Salvarsan was later followed by Neosalvarsan (which was less dangerous to the patient than Salvarsan had been),[34] and once it became better known, it was the preferred treatment for syphilis, even in the colonies.

Salvarsan arrived in most of the colonies in 1911. In 1910/11, Dr. Rodenwaldt reported that starting the follow year he planned to use Salvarsan in conjunction with potassium iodide to treat syphilis, which he did with apparent success. In that same year, reports from Cameroon indicated that it was also being used there.[35] Physicians in DSWA began using it to treat syphilitic patients in Windhoek—both European and indigenous—in January 1911. The following month it was used in Keetmanshoop. The chief medical officer for the colony, Dr. Mayer, stated that it "enjoys here in the short time of [its] use the same recognition in terms of prompt effectiveness and surprising successes it does in Europe."[36] Doctors in the Pacific also commented on its efficacy. In 1911/12, one government physician spoke of its "beneficial effects" in fighting syphilis.[37] Dr. Meyer on Truk (in the Caroline Islands) noted that of the "115 Salvarsan injections" he "carried out" "in order to save people's lives and to prevent the worst dangers," "almost all of them" were completely successful.[38]

Though it initially had been hailed as a "magic bullet," only its ability to cure syphilis had been established, not its overall efficacy and suitability. In other words, many questions still remained, such as the correct dosage and the best means of administering it, before it could become an established fact that Salvarsan was truly the "one-shot cure."[39] In professional journals, physicians shared their clinical experiences and debated how best to proceed with Salvarsan. Meanwhile, opponents of the new cure pointed to the serious side effects of it and the possibility that a Salvarsan treatment could result in death.[40] The lively discussions surrounding Salvarsan were closely connected to the issue of human experimentation and the changing doctor-patient relationship.

Although guidelines existed in Prussia since 1900 regarding research with patients in Prussian hospitals, these were apparently not followed during the clinical trials for Salvarsan. Rather, as in previous instances with human test subjects, those most often selected as test subjects were those that were at the margins in German society, and thus did not possess any real voice or agency. These included children, prostitutes, or the insane (*Geisteskranke*). Physicians at that time believed in the power of science to change the world and experimentation was necessary to further scientific knowledge that would benefit all of humanity. Thus, doctors and scientists did not need to ask their patients (especially those that were not a part of mainstream society anyway) because only they possessed the scientific training and knowledge as demonstrated through their state sanctioned and professionally required exams to know what was best for the patient, a position that German society increasingly acceded to them.[41]

The use of Salvarsan in the colonies was closely associated with resolving many of the unanswered questions connected to the new medication. Often, the colonies were testing grounds for new medicines, though primarily in Africa. This was facilitated by the racial inequality that characterized the colonial situation, which placed Africans at the bottom of the racial hierarchy. Like those who were often the objects of experiments in Germany, Africans were politically marginalized and were perceived as being less capable of knowing what was best for them. In other words, because of their medical and racial objectification, colonial physicians felt justified in using indigenes as test subjects in the search for new medicines and treatments, especially for those diseases that threatened the colonial economy, such as sleeping sickness.[42]

With specific regards to Salvarsan, many colonial physicians actively participated in furthering the research on Salvarsan as part of the larger effort of advancing scientific knowledge. While not exclusive to Africa, doctors there often tested Salvarsan on indigenous patients not only to combat the spread of VD, but also to gather medical information for later use in the homeland.[43] In DSWA, the use of Salvarsan was limited to the hospitals in Windhoek and Keetmanshoop, where the attending physicians were ordered to keep an exact log "so that later a summary report [could] be submitted to the Imperial Colonial Office."[44] Dr. Seibert tested for the best way to administer Salvarsan at the "native" hospital in Winhoek. After first trying the intramuscular method, he rejected it because "without exception it resulted in tissue necrosis (*Gewebsnekrosen*) the size of fists, which had to be treated for months before they healed." He then tried the intravenous method, which was "extraordinarily" successful. He shared his findings in the 1910/11 edition of the *Medizinal-Berichte,* where he reported in a matter of fact manner that "the injection is almost painless, without damage to the place of injection, the effect is speedy and certain. Already after 8 days obvious success, even for a native conclusive."[45] Similarly, in the 1911/12 report for DOA, there was an entire section devoted to the use of Salvarsan in the colony. One contributor, Dr. Neubert, shared that after first using the intramuscular means of administering the drug, he then utilized the intravenous method because he found that it worked "faster and more resoundingly" than the first method.[46]

The colonies also became a place to test the ability of this chemotherapeutic compound to cure other illnesses. The primary focus was on various bacteria that Hata and Ehrlich grouped together in their 1910 book, *Experimentelle Chemotherapie der Spirillosen (Syphilis, Rückfallfieber, Hühnerspirillose, Frambösie)* (The Experimental Chemotherapy of Spirilloses [Syphilis, Relapsing Fever, Spirillosis of fowls, Framboesia]).[47] In this book, the two detailed their observations from their experiments on animals. In the colonial setting, various colonial doctors took Hata and Ehrlich's work to the next level by using Salvarsan to treat not just syphilis, but these other illnesses as well. For example, in reports from East Africa, several doctors detailed their use of the arsenic compound to treat these various diseases, including how they administered Salvarsan, the dosage, and the frequency of the drug's use. Dr. Grothusen in his report noted that one German woman treated with Salvarsan for relapsing fever had no more attacks while another one who did not receive Salvarsan treatments had four additional attacks.[48] In the Pacific, physicians spoke of their success in fighting yaws with the drug.[49]

Like their counterparts at home, doctors utilized disciplinary measures based on scientific knowledge and bourgeois conceptions of health and race. The success of these efforts depended in large part on surveillance tactics. More than their colleagues in Germany, the colonial situation enabled physicians to require broader segments of the population to submit to medical examinations. In addition, they required those found infected to undergo treatment until cured, essentially using imprisonment in some instances. Through the use of such tactics, colonial doctors believed that they had made some headway in fighting the spread of VD, but they also conceded that they still had a lot of work to do. Both depended on indigenous behavior, which at times prompted physicians to modify how they interacted with non-Europeans or to resort to more punitive steps.

Notes

1. *MB 1903/04* (1905): 243.
2. *MB 1909/10* (1911): 506; Imperial Governor, DOA, to all departments on the coast, 8 March 1901, 56–57. See also Levine, *Prostitution, Race and Politics,* 67.
3. Born, Die gesundheitliche Verhältnisse auf dem Atoll Ebon, November 1913, 30.
4. Ibid.
5. *MB 1907/08* (1909): 356.
6. *MB 1910/11* (1913): 796.
7. Sauerteig, *Krankheit, Sexualität, Gesellschaft,* 33; and Oriel, *The Scars of Venus,* 77–80.
8. Heim, "Die Syphilis in den deutschen Schutzgebieten," 170–171; and Jäger, "Beiträge zur Rassenhygiene," 334; Karen Jochelson, "Tracking Down the Treponema: Patterns of Syphilis in South Africa, 1880–1940," STRUCTURE AND EXPERIENCE IN THE MAKING OF APARTHEID, History Workshop, University of Witwatersrand; accessed through WIReDSpace, University of Witwatersrand, Johannesburg, 2002–2011, http://wiredspace.wits.ac.za/bitstream/handle/10539/7881/HWS-202.pdf?sequence=1 (accessed 12 April 2012); Oriel, *Scars of Venus,* 75–76.
9. *MB 1910/11* (1913): 493.
10. Born, Die gesundheitliche Verhältnisse auf dem Atoll Ebon, November 1913, 30.
11. For example, see Mense, "Syphilis und venerische Krankheiten," 88. See also Heim, "Die Syphilis in den deutschen Schutzgebieten," 165–198.
12. *MB 1907/08* (1909): 201.
13. Heim, "Die Syphilis in den deutschen Schutzgebieten," 191, 196–198; Scheube, "Die venerischen Krankheiten in den warmen Ländern," *ASTH* 6, no. 5 (1902): 147–160; Scheube, "Die venerischen Krankheiten in den warmen Ländern (Fortseztung)," 187–207; Scheube, "Die venerischen Krankheiten in den warmen Ländern (Fortsetzung und Schluss)," 219–244, especially 241; and Hugo Zechmeister, "Die Syphilis in den Tropen, deren Verlauf und Behandlung," *ASTH* 12, no. 11 (1908): 350–351.
14. *MB 1909/10* (1911): 328. See also Rechenberg, Governor German East Africa, Verfügung betr. Geschlechtskrankheiten, 1 December 1910, BArch R1001/6040, 136.
15. *MB 1906/07* (1908): 172.

16. Dr. Philipp Goos, "Bubo" Jameda, 2007–2012, last update 2 March 2012, http://www.jameda.de/medikamente/krankheiten/tropischer-bubo/a55_4209/ (accessed 11 April 2012).
17. *MB 1905/06* (1907): 437.
18. Ibid., 82.
19. *MB 1903/04* (1905): 243.
20. Ibid., 243.
21. *MB 1904/05* (1907): 172.
22. *MB 1906/07* (1908): 227.
23. *MB 1910/11* (1913): 647.
24. *MB 1911/12* (1915): 520.
25. For the colonial experience, see *MB 1905/06* (1907): 419; *MB 1906/07* (1908): 57; *MB 1908/09* (1910): 215; *MB 1910/11* (1913): 647; *MB 1911/12* (1915): 521. For a more complete description of how males were treated in Germany, see Oriel, *The Scars of Venus,* 140–144.
26. *MB 1908/09* (1910): 66. See also MB *1907/08* (1909): 78.
27. Santyl later became used as a topical, not internal, medicine used to treat various skin ailments.
28. *MB 1906/07* (1908): 57.
29. *MB 1908/09* (1910): 215.
30. Oriel, *The Scars of Venus,* 144.
31. Ibid.
32. Ibid., 144–145, 141–142.
33. *MB 1903/04* (1905): 73; MB *1904/05* (1907): 46, 218; *MB 1905/06* (1907): 80–81, 263; *MB 1906/07* (1908): 241; *MB 1907/08* (1909): 82; *MB 1908/09* (1910): 66, 511; *MB 1909/10* (1911): 506, 577; *MB 1910/*11 (1913): 647, 719. See also Oriel, *The Scars of Venus,* 86–89; Sauerteig, *Krankheit, Sexualität, Gesellschaft,* 34.
34. Lutz Sauerteig, "Salvarsan und der 'ärztliche Polizeistaat,'" 163–169; Sauerteig *Krankheit, Sexualität, Gesellschaft,* 34; Oriel, *The Scars of Venus,* 89–93; Axel Hüntelmann, "1910. Transformationen eines Arzneistoffes—vom 606 zum Salvarsan," in *Arzneimittel des 20. Jahrhunderts: 13 historische Skizzen von Lebertran bis Contergan,* ed. N. Eschenbruch et al. (Bielefeld: Transcript, 2009), 17–51.
35. *MB 1910/11* (1913): 493; *MB 1911/12* (1915): 441, 421.
36. *MB 1910/11* (1913): 588. See also *MB 1910/11* (1913): 795.
37. *MB 1911/12* (1915): 588.
38. Meyer, Medical Report, 30 September 1913, Truk, NAA G2/U17, 52–55.
39. For more on this concept of what constitutes a scientific fact, see Ludwik Fleck, *Genesis and Development of a Scientific Fact* (Chicago: University of Chicago Press, 1979).
40. Oriel, *The Scars of Venus,* 92–93; Sauerteig, "Salvarsan und der 'ärztliche Polizeistaat,'" 166–169. See also the many essays in Paul Ehrlich, ed., *Abhandlungen über Salvarsan (Ehrlich-Hata Präparat 606) gegen Syphilis* (Munich: J.F. Lehmann's Verlag, 1911); Wilhelm Wechselmann, *The Treatment of Syphilis with Salvarsan,* trans. Abraham Wolbarst (New York: Rebman, 1911).
41. Lutz Sauerteig, "Ethische Richtlinien," 303–334; Elkeles, *Der moralische Diskurs,* 2–5, 225–231. For a detailed discussion of human experimentation within the field of venereology, see Elke Tashiro, *Die Waage des Venus: Venerologische Versuche am Menschen zwischen Fortschritt und Moral* (Husum: Matthiesen Verlag, 1991).
42. Elkeles, *Der moralische Diskurs,* 229–230; Wolfgang Eckart, "Arzneimittelerprobung in der ehemaligen deutschen Kolonie Togo," *Forum Wissenschaft* 1 (1988): 29–35; Neill, "Transnationalism," 328–329; Isobe, *Medizin und Kolonialismus,* 91–118, 178–201, 238–265; Hüntelmann, "1910," 21.
43. Oermann, *Mission, Church and State Relations,* 11; Hahl, Imperial Governor, to Regierungsarzt in Jaluit, 12 September 1912, NAA G2/U24, 16.
44. Seitz to Imperial District Offices, 1 March 1911, BArch R151F/H.ii.H.3: 21.
45. *MB 1910/11* (1913): 588.

46. *MB 1911/12* (1915): 209.
47. Paul Ehrlich and Sahachiro Hata, *Experimentelle Chemotherapie der Spirillosen (Syphilis, Rückfallfieber, Hühnerspirillose, Frambösie)* (Berlin: Springer, 1910).
48. *MB 1911/12* (1915): 208–215, especially 209.
49. *MB 1911/12* (1915): 588–589; Born, Die gesundheitliche Verhältnisse auf dem Atoll Ebon, November 1913, 30.

Chapter 10

Assessing the Surveillance

Throughout the period of German colonial control, especially in the twentieth century, physicians reported and commented on the programs they implemented and their efficacy in their campaign to stop the spread of venereal diseases. They remarked on the effectiveness of certain policies, while simultaneously pointing out where work needed to be done. By the end of colonial rule, however, while they could point to a number of successes, overall they believed that they still had a lot of work to do.

According to some reports, initially it appeared that the various surveillance and treatment measures to fight VD were having some impact. Already in 1902/03, even before knowledge about the origins of syphilis and the availability of the Wassermann test, Dr. Meixner reported that the steps taken in East Africa along the coast in Tabora had already resulted in some early success, at least in protecting Europeans. In the following year, Dr. Schörnich wrote that among the African soldiers, the controls did lead to a reduction in the number of recorded incidents.[1] By 1911/12, Dr. Exner in Dar es Salaam noted that "venereal diseases in [the city] have generally declined through the regular examinations of the [prostitute]; acute syphilis cases have become seldom."[2]

Officials in other colonies also noted that the required examinations of service personnel and others were contributing to the decline in the number of infected persons. For instance, in Douala (Cameroon), only twenty-eight cases among African soldiers were reported in 1908/09, which Dr. Ziemann described as "a very favorable success." Colony-wide, the number of African soldiers infected with VD started to decline in the two years after 1906/07 (see appendix, table 5). Dr. Ziemann explained that the positive results were "achieved through

Notes for this section begin on page 119.

the diligent examination of the soldiers and their followers [i.e., their wives] as well as the compulsory treatment of prostitutes by the government physician."[3] In DSWA, a physician writing in the 1911/12 General Sanitary Report for the Imperial Colonial Troops remarked that the use of condoms by soldiers was "an essential preventive."[4]

Similarly, the measures were having an apparent impact on German colonial troops. In Cameroon, for instance, venereal infections remained consistently low among German soldiers (see appendix, table 5). In Qingdao, the chief naval officer, Dr. Hans Podestà, reported a much-improved situation among German military personnel. Writing in 1909, he commented that since 1900/01 the number of infected soldiers had decreased every year to the point that it now occurred less frequently than in the regular navy, sinking from a morbidity rate of 26.06 percent in 1900/01 to 4.15 percent in 1906/07 (see appendix, table 18). He attributed the success to "good supervision of the prostitution, instruction, and prophylaxis of venereal diseases."[5]

Moreover, numerous examples existed of more people either submitting to medical examinations or staying in treatment until healed. For example, among "coloreds" in the New Guinea Old Protectorate, the number of infected in treatment (and ultimately those healed) increased throughout the colonial period, a situation fairly common throughout the overseas territories (see appendix, table 13 for DNG, table 3 for Cameroon, table 6 for DSWA, and table 9 for DOA).

Not only did the number of patients in treatment increase over time, but also the percentage of those completing their cure. For instance, in 1904/05 DOA, the lowest percentage of registered patients healed (82 percent) was recorded. In the following years, though, the percentage increased, reaching 89 percent in 1911/12.[6] Some of the other colonies had similar experiences (e.g., see appendix, table 1 for Togo, table 3 for Cameroon, and table 13 for the DNG Old Protectorate). It should, though, be noted that the healed rate for the last recorded year was not always the highest rate for tabulated years (e.g., see appendix, table 9).

Moreover, statistics, though problematic, did reveal that most autochthons completed their treatment, while those who left were almost always a minority. Between 1903/04 and 1909/10, only an average of 10 percent of African patients in East Africa did not complete their treatment (with the medium being 9 percent), while for the same period the average for those finishing their cures was 84.7 percent (and a medium of 85 percent).[7] In Samoa, officials reported a 100 percent cure rate in both 1910/11 and 1911/12 for registered "colored" and "Chinese" as well as "European patients," the highest percentage recorded for the colony (see appendix, table 16).

Admittedly, in many colonies doctors reported increases in the number of VD cases over the years. However, one physician in DOA attributed the rise to increased control and not necessarily due to its spread, at least among soldiers. Dr. Meixner, writing in 1910/11, remarked that the "number of new cases of venereal diseases" played only a "subordinate role." He stated that "the increase in morbidity is only an apparent one, it is caused only by the stricter supervision that was introduced everywhere."[8]

From the perspective of colonial doctors, not only did increased surveillance methods contribute to the decline in VD, but also ostensibly to changes in indigenous behavior. For these doctors, those who sought and agreed to European treatments indicated that these people did embrace or at least adopt Western medicine and public health education. In German New Guinea, for example, a local doctor noted that "the free natives more and more call on the European physician in order to be treated by him."[9] A similar situation existed in parts of DSWA, where more Africans requested treatment for VD "on their own accord."[10] A colonial doctor in Douala stated that recently "fathers-in-law sent their future sons-in-law to the doctor before the weddings for the purpose of being examined for venereal disease." He described this as "a happy (*erfreuliche*) result of the public health instructions held for coloreds."[11] Meanwhile, his colleague in Kribi, Cameroon, reported that "because the danger of infection from gonorrhea *appears* [*scheint*; emphasis added] to be known, a certain amount of protection is exercised by the natives themselves," which resulted in a decline in the number of gonorrhea infections.[12]

However, as Gwyn Prins has pointed out, non-Europeans already possessed knowledge of health and disease prior to the arrival of the Europeans. The behavior, therefore, was more a demonstration of continuity than a change in indigenous medicine.[13] In fact, even German doctors admitted that prior to their arrival in the colonies, indigenous cultures did possess an understanding of illness and health.[14] Dr. Grothusen in Bukoba District (DOA) remarked that "the natives have an astonishing knowledge of the disease [i.e., syphilis]." He noted that "almost every day sick people come to the polyclinic, who complain about chest pain, specify syphilis as the reason and request potassium iodide."[15]

Thus, though their direct voice was largely absent from colonial records, indigenes quite plausibly recognized the dangers of VD and saw the advantages in seeking medical assistance. This was certainly evident in the case of the Cameroonian fathers. They pursued such actions not necessarily in open support of German public health agendas, but rather out of their own self-interests. Therefore, in all probability many sought treatment and completed it simply because they wanted to, which may or may not have been an indication of some subjectification occurring in the colonial environment.

This most likely applied to some prostitutes in East Africa and Togo. They may have willingly submitted to examinations and treatments in order to be allowed to conduct their business. In these colonies, officials required those women registered as prostitutes to carry a card or book that indicated their current state of health and most recent examination.[16] According to Dr. Liebl in Lomé, Togo, "this card already represents for prostitutes quite a coveted and valuable object,"[17] which may have been true for some women.[18]

This apparent willingness to go to German doctors may also have been a result of increased trust in German doctors and medicine. Indeed, how German doctors interacted with non-European patients may have had an impact on indigenous perceptions of both them and their treatments. As a matter of fact, colonial health authorities recognized that this was important if they were to succeed[19]—and some were apparently successful. For instance, Dr. Born on Truk in the Pacific reported that his predecessor Dr. Meyer had "paved the way exceptionally well, the people have trust in the doctor and follow willingly all directions."[20]

The efficacy of treatments may have acted as an incentive for individuals to seek treatment and contributed to limiting the impact of VD. Doctors in Windhoek (DSWA) believed this to be the case. In a study on the need for a "native" hospital (*Eingeborenen Lazarett*) in the colonial capital, the local physician remarked that the best way to convince Africans to come willingly to the hospital was by curing them of their ailments, including venereal diseases. He argued that African confidence in European medicine accounted for the increased frequency of Africans coming freely to German doctors for treatments.[21]

German physicians maintained a similar perspective after the introduction of Salvarsan into the colonial environment. Dr. Mayer on Ponape (East Carolines) stated:

> The sufficiently proven beneficial effect of Salvarsan had found here a large field for application. Syphilis and yaws were treated in the past 2 months in almost 100 cases, with almost always complete success, complications occurred almost never or only temporarily. The success is best demonstrated by the fact that a girl, who was already 6 years in the hospital with syphilis in treatment, after 4 weeks, and a woman, who lived eight months with the same disease in the hospital, with only 14 days after treatment with Salvarsan could be discharged as cured. The often numerous and wide-spread ulcers healed quickly and with good scarring under simple Vaseline application.[22]

His colleague in East Africa went so far as to say that "the people had great trust in the 'new remedy' and came in great numbers in order to receive the Salvarsan injection."[23]

The fact that medicine was provided for free to indigenes may have acted as an incentive for many to seek out a German doctor. Indeed, increasingly throughout the colonial empire, authorities saw the provision of free medicine as a means both to encourage non-Europeans to visit German doctors and to promote public health policies. In German New Guinea, for instance, the policy was to give Pacific Islanders and Asians free medicine unless they were employed directly by a private company.[24] In Southwest Africa, the district officer in Okahndja believed that the provision of free medicine to Africans "would be in the interest of the reputation of the young institution [the 'native hospital'] as well as in the interest of their employers, for whom the labor of the natives would otherwise be missing for a longer time."[25] Dr. Mayer reported that since the Southwest African government assumed the cost for treating VD, "a much higher admittance [*Zugang*] of venereal patients to native hospitals" has occurred.[26]

While it may not have a direct role in encouraging patients to visit a physician, the growth in medical personnel and the expansion of medical facilities did nonetheless enhance health officials' ability to bring more individuals under surveillance. Between 1884 and 1914, approximately 550 civilian and military physicians worked in Germany's overseas territories. Most of these (339 of them) served in the military. Of the remaining 211 civilian doctors, 145 were directly employed by the Colonial Department of the Foreign Office (after 1907 the Imperial Colonial Office, or RKA). The others either worked for the various missionary societies (36) or for different companies (30).[27]

In addition, other medical personnel were employed in the colonies, including nurses from the German Women's Association for Nursing in the Colonies, military medics, and other lay individuals with basic medical training. The latter often included both male and female indigenes. The training of indigenous health personnel was intended to offset the dearth in German medical personnel. Their presence was also intended to make other indigenes more comfortable in seeking out German medical knowledge.[28] Within the context of combating VD, the government in East Africa requested that the Imperial Colonial Office send a female physician to the territory. The government in Dar es Salaam recognized that African women were "in general completely" averse to "a treatment or an examination by a male doctor for genital diseases." As the campaign against malaria demonstrated, "female personnel are extraordinarily beneficial in this work." Consequently, the RKA supported the request, but was not especially confident it could find someone appropriate for the task.[29]

Further, during the German colonial period, the number of hospitals and clinics serving both Europeans and non-Europeans also increased, though primarily to the benefit of whites. In DSWA, by the end of the colonial period, there were seventeen hospitals that served the white population (eleven public, six private) in places like Windhoek and Swakopmund as well as facilities for the military. Moreover, there were two public hospitals (Lüderitz Bay and Swakopmund) and other facilities in Windhoek, Okahandja, Keetmanshoop, and elsewhere. In West Africa, Togo had two hospitals for Europeans and two for Africans, while in Cameroon racially segregated facilities for both whites and Africans existed in Douala, Victoria, and Kribi. In addition, there were several infirmaries located throughout Cameroon in places such as Edea, Jaunde, and Kusseri.[30]

In German East Africa, there were two main hospitals for Europeans (Dar es Salaam and Tanga), plus a number of infirmaries stationed close to white settlements. A number of these infirmaries grew into medium-sized hospitals. In addition, some of them also began to serve Africans. The only major hospital for non-Europeans, the Sewa Hadij Hospital, was located in colonial capital. Another one existed in Tanga.[31]

In the Pacific, there were a variety of facilities located throughout Germany's possessions. For example, in New Guinea there were government hospitals for Europeans in Herbertshöhe and Namanula near Rabaul as well as a polyclinic in Herbertshöhe. Facilities also existed on Jaluit and Nauru in the Marshall Islands and on Yap and Ponape in the Caroline Islands. For non-Europeans, there were hospitals in Herbertshöhe, Simpsonhafen, Rabaul, as well as on Nauru and

Jaluit. Facilities were also established on Yap and Ponape. Moreover, numerous private facilities existed for most of the contract labor. In fact, private hospitals and clinics had more beds than government hospitals. Apia on Samoa had a public hospital for both Europeans and non-European (with separate rooms).[32] On the Chinese mainland in Kiautschou, numerous facilities existed for the German military personnel. In addition, the Germans built a hospital for prostitutes and ran several polyclinics for the Chinese population.[33]

When health officials cited examples of indigenes embracing Western medical knowledge, this was an ostensible indication that a certain degree of subjectification was occurring. Such instances included the Cameroonian fathers-in-law and the patients in the Bukoba district, but overall they were given little space in the documents. When they reported such incidents, they often used such language as "happy" and "appears,"[34] suggesting either surprise in the former case or skepticism in the latter. In these cases, were Africans truly capable of following German health instructions? As Megan Vaughan has argued, such behavior on the part of Africans "was interpreted [by Europeans] as evidence of their continuing belief in 'magic.'"[35] While not exactly the same in these cases, the comments revealed perhaps a persistence of racial stereotyping, for they suggested that such behavior was extraordinary. In fact, the same physician in Kribi (Cameroon), who remarked that some Africans were aware of the dangers of venereal infection, ultimately concluded that their other racial characteristics prevented them from keeping themselves and those around them in a state of health. He wrote that "one can naturally speak less in Africa than in Europe from a purposeful campaign against venereal diseases."[36]

Notes

1. *AkG* (1904): 567; *MB 1905/06* (1907): 364.
2. *MB 1911/12* (1915): 170.
3. *MB 1908/09* (1910): 510–511.
4. *MB 1911/12* (1915): 655.
5. Podestà, "Entwicklung und Gestaltung," 589, 584, 576.
6. Calculations based on the figures provided in appendix, table 9.
7. Calculations based on the figures provided in appendix, table 9.
8. *MB 1910/11* (1913): 756.
9. Aerztlicher Bericht über die Zeit vom 1 July–30 September 1909, 16 October 1909, BArch R1001/5771, 187; Rechenberg, Runderlass an Sanitätsdienststellen und Regierungsärzte, 24 August 1911, BArch R1001/5671, 127.
10. Denkschrift zur Bekämpfung der Geschlechtskrankheiten, 5 November 1908, 21–22. See also Wohlgemuth to Imperial Government in Windhoek, 30 May 1911, BArch R151F/H.ii.H.3.
11. Medizinalbericht für Kamerun 1909/10, 1910, BArch R1001/6012, 1.
12. Ibid.

13. Gwyn Prins, "Review Article: But what was the disease? The present state of health and healing in African Studies," *Past and Present* 124 (1989): 159–179. See also Vaughan, *Curing their Ills,* 24.
14. Protokoll über die Besprechung des Gouverneurs mit den Vorleuten der Eingeborenen, Windhoek, 17 October 1908, BArch R1001/6040, 25–28; Medical Office, DSWA, Denkschrift zur Bekämpfung der Geschlechtskrankheiten, 8 November 1908, 21–22.
15. *MB 1910/11* (1913): 86.
16. Imperial Governor to all departments on the coast, 8 March 1901, 56; *MB 1911/12* (1915): 173; *MB 07/08* (1909): 251; *MB 1911/12* (1915): 173.
17. *MB 07/08* (1909): 251.
18. Imperial Governor, DOA, to all departments on the coast, 8 March 1901, BArch R1001/5745, 56.
19. See for example the comments of the Dr. Wolff in Lindi (DOA), *MB 1911/12* (1915): 171.
20. Dr. Born, Medical Report, 4 March 1914, NAA G2/U17, 61–63.
21. Vorschläge zur Errichting eines massiven Eingeborenenlazaretts in Windhuk, 1908, BArch R1001/6042, 10.
22. *MB 1911/12* (1915): 588.
23. Exner, Bericht über die gesundheitlichen Verhältnisse in Deutsch-Ostafrika in der Zeit vom 1 January–31 March 1914, 1914, BArch R1001/5747, 254.
24. Johannes Grüntzig and Heinz Mehlhorn, *Expeditionen ins Reich der Seuchen: Medizinische Himmelsfahrtskommando der deutschen Kaiser- und Kolonialzeit* (Munich: Spektrum, 2005), 49; Aerztlicher Bericht über die Zeit vom 1 April–30 June 1909, Rabaul, 16 July 1909, BArch R1001/5771, 128–132.
25. Distriktamtmann to Imperial Government in Windhoek, 6 December 1912, BAB R151F/H. ii.h.i., 97.
26. *MB 1910/11* (1913): 586–587.
27. Eckart, *Medizin und Kolonialimperialismus,* 118–119; Eckart, "Medicine and German colonial expansion," 80–102, especially 81–84.
28. Eckart, *Medizin und Kolonialismus,* 10, 41–55, 129, 148, 152, 156, 158, 177, 179, 184, 200, 212–214, 232, 238, 351, 353, 357, 365, 379, 381 391, 395, 398, 418, 426–427, 432–433, 446–447, 449, 453, 503, 531.
29. RKA to Dr. Petzold, 13 March 1913, BArch R1001/5962, 143.
30. Eckart, *Medizin und Kolonialismus,* 260, 134–145, 196–201.
31. Ibid., 315–318.
32. Ibid., 394, 421–427, 433, 435, 448.
33. Ibid., 469–471, 475–478, 478–480, 481–482.
34. Medizinalbericht für Kamerun 1909/10, 1910, 1.
35. Vaughan, *Curing their Ills,* 151.
36. Medizinalbericht für Kamerun 1909/10, 1910, 1.

Chapter 11

Perceived Ongoing Challenges

While some German doctors agreed that progress was being made, others believed that venereal diseases continued to pose a threat. In fact, as in other European colonies[1] and even in Germany,[2] colonial physicians viewed the various measures pursued as insufficient because the diseases continued to spread and the number of infected ostensibly rose. For instance, even though Dr. Ziemann spoke of a decrease in venereal infections in 1908/09, he noted that African soldiers in Cameroon continued to become infected while traveling on patrols into the interior. He pointed out that then the infection would again be "transferred to the entire station garrison, because the soldiers' wives almost without exception engage in prostitution."[3] He also wrote that this contributed to the wives' infertility,[4] a reference to the concern about the future existence of a colonized people that could serve their German "masters." In 1913, his successor reported that in Ngaundere, "the entire population is apparently completely contaminated with sexually transmitted diseases of every type."[5] Similarly in German New Guinea, Dr. Born spoke of "a catastrophic spread of syphilis" on the atoll Arno.[6]

A similar situation also existed among the white population. In Southwest Africa (DSWA), Dr. Schelle reported that with regards to white colonial soldiers, "all instructions, health examinations, the dissemination of leaflets and prophylaxes were without result."[7] In East Africa, where earlier reports indicated that advances had been made, the situation had apparently deteriorated by 1905/06. In his annual report from that year, the colonial physician wrote that "among the Europeans [venereal diseases] have nearly doubled, despite the examination of prostitutes."[8]

Notes for this section begin on page 129.

Statistical evidence appeared to support these assertions in many of the overseas territories. Thus, while numbers were declining in places like Qingdao and Samoa, in most other places VD cases appeared to be on the rise despite the various measures. In East Africa, for instance, the number of reported cases among Africans more than doubled for the period from 1903/04 to 1911/12, going from 996 to 2,650 in the final reporting year (see appendix, table 10). In Togo after 1908/09, the number of African cases began to decline steadily, only to rise again in the final reporting year to above three hundred (see appendix, table 1). Meanwhile in Cameroon, the number of reported patients for both "Europeans" and "coloreds" rose over the years. For whites, the figure more than doubled in the last reported year (1911/12) over the previous one, jumping from 71 to 154 (see appendix, table 3). A similar increase was also statistically indicated in DSWA among whites and Africans, though the evidence was reported inconsistently (see appendix, table 6). In German New Guinea, in both the Old Protectorate and in the Island Territories, the number of cases in general rose over the years (see appendix, table 13), though in some districts the figures actually dropped (see appendix, table 14).

As previously stated, some doctors saw an increase in the number of registered patients as an indication that certain policies were working. The significant increase in recorded cases for the New Guinea Island Territories in 1911/12 suggested that some of the measures may have worked particularly well that year. Others, though, argued that the statistics did not provide an accurate assessment of the full extent of venereal contamination. Dr. Mayer noted that in DSWA there was a "tremendous spread of sexually transmitted diseases … among natives" in 1910/11, which was not objectively represented in "quantitative documents."[9]

Moreover, some of those who were diagnosed with VD left treatment before it was completed. For example, of the 468 indigenous cases initially treated for gonorrhea in East Africa in 1904/05, 56 were reported as "elsewhere (*anderweitig*)," implying they were no longer under German supervision. With regard to syphilis cases, 5 of the initial 26 cases were also reported as "elsewhere."[10] In Togo, over 20 percent of Africans diagnosed with VD did not complete their treatment. In 1908/09 and 1909/10, the figure rose to 32 percent and 33 percent respectively (percentages based on figures in appendix, table 1). Hence, while often the number of patients who were cured usually rose, those who did not complete their treatment still remained problematic for the campaign.

The percentages for Europeans were often even higher. In Cameroon, for instance, over 50 percent of whites were categorized as "elsewhere" in 1908/09 (figure based on statistics from appendix, table 3). In Togo, the figures ranged from as low as 13 percent in 1908/09 (with incomplete data) to 38 percent in the following year (percentages based on data in appendix, table 1). Europeans in East Africa consistently had a higher percentage of infected in the "elsewhere" category than Africans. For Africans, the highest percentage was 14 percent in 1905/06, while for Europeans it was 35 percent in 1908/09. The lowest figures for Europeans were 13 percent and 14 percent recorded in 1905/06 and 1906/07 respectively. However, these were exceptions. Normally the figure was above 20 percent (based on data compiled in appendix, table 9).

A similar situation existed in German New Guinea. In both the Old Protectorate and the Island Territories, the percentage of Europeans categorized as "elsewhere" was repeatedly larger than "coloreds." In the Old Protectorate, the figure was normally above 10 percent, reaching as high as 24 percent in 1909/10. In the Island Territories, the lowest figure was 18 percent in 1908/09, but in most years it was well above 20 percent. Admittedly, in both locations the total number of cases was relatively small (calculations based on data in appendix, table 13). The fear was that those who left before being cured would engage in sexual intercourse and consequently contribute to further spreading VD.[11]

Because of these apparent problems with individuals leaving before their treatment was completed, and hence continuing to pose a health risk, special facilities were created. As one official in Cameroon stated, "as long as they [Africans] are on the loose, they do not take care of their illness."[12] One response was to treat women in a special section of a "native" hospital. Another was to build special barracks for prostitutes where they were to be treated. Over time, even some of these structures proved insufficient, as evidenced by the addition of fences to some buildings to keep the patients interned until risk free.[13] In many British colonies, such as India, Hong Kong, and Australia, so-called lock hospitals served a similar function and were more ubiquitous.[14]

In East Africa, the government even set up a syphilis camp (*Krankenlager*) on the island of Ukerewe in Lake Victoria. The camp was under the direction of Dr. Petzoldt and its main aim was to combat the different forms of syphilis and yaws prevalent on the island. It also collected data on the use of Salvarsan and the Wassermann reaction.[15] Hence, it was similar to the camps established to fight sleeping sickness in German East Africa, Togo, and Cameroon, where new drugs were tested on individuals who did not have a choice and were contained in enclosed spaces.[16] On Ukerewe, there was no fence, but it was an island, which made it easier to identify and control the infected population. Dr. Born wanted to establish something similar in the Pacific. However, unlike the East African camp, the small atoll would be used to send all those in the region infected with gonorrhea to be "effectively treated and isolated."[17] From the documentary record, it was not clear if his request was fulfilled.

The existence of these German facilities, though, offered no guarantee that patients would complete their treatment. As early as 1896, Dr. Becker in East Africa reported that it was nearly impossible to keep infected African soldiers in the military hospital. "Also the situation that the interaction of the 'colored military hospital' with the outside world cannot be prevented contributes to the spread of venereal diseases. Not infrequently do the infected leave the hospital at night and infect their own or also other women during their nightly excursions. The potential penalties in case of discovery only seldom deter the coloreds endowed with an active sex drive."[18] Nearly two decades later, Dr. Born expressed similar complaints about indigenous behavior in the Pacific, despite the existence of a fence and then later armed guards:

> After the previous experience it would not be appropriate to treat all the sick in the Jabwor hospital. Despite all supervision the venereally infected from Ebon have had the opportunity to have sex both amongst themselves as well as with those outside [the hospital]. It has even transpired that a woman infected with gonorrhea has dug under the fence in order to get outside! After the imperial station provided police soldiers to increase supervision, the infected girls took up even with these in the night. An ordered investigation did not bring out the least results, because all the girls stated that they had been constantly harassed by the soldiers at night.[19]

For these physicians, both incidents illustrated that additional work was needed to stop the spread of venereal diseases as a result of the apparent licentious behavior of the indigenes. Indeed, such reports appeared to reaffirm physicians' perceptions of non-European sexuality.

Government doctors noted several reasons for these setbacks. One frequently mentioned factor was the lack of sufficient funds. Indeed, throughout the colonial era, the colonies experienced budgetary constraints from the Reichstag (the German parliament), which controlled all aspects of colonial administration related to expenditures. While the Reichstag had allocated approximately 646 million marks in subsides for the colonies between 1884 and 1914, many requests went unfunded, even after the advent of the Dernburg Era and the greater emphasis on promoting the health and welfare of indigenes. This was due to the fact that most budgetary discussions, even those relating to colonial issues, were really about domestic issues and the Reichstag (or groups in it) trying to assert itself against the imperial government.[20]

Consequently, this made it difficult to supply enough public health officials or medicine or to construct the proper facilities to meet the challenges associated with fighting the proliferation of VD. According to Dr. Born in the South Seas, "Unfortunately at this time the medical activity is to a large degree hampered by the scarcity of many necessary medicines as well as through the lack of a primitive hospital. For the medical practice only a pitiful hut next to the prison is available, which is entirely inadequate."[21] In addition, by the beginning of 1914, there were only 139 physicians throughout Germany's overseas possessions, which included approximately 14 million inhabitants. Thus, there was one doctor for every 100,000 "potential patients." This was even after Colonial Secretary Bernhard Dernburg made a concerted effort to improve indigenous health conditions after 1907.[22]

Closely tied to the deficiency in personnel and facilities was the reality of examining all targeted groups and maintaining control over the infected—i.e., exercising jurisdiction over a significantly larger population living in vast regions or, in the case of the Pacific, scattered territories.[23] For instance, authorities complained that it was increasingly difficult to register all prostitutes because many engaged in what is known as opportunity prostitution.[24] In Lomé, Togo, one doctor reported that "through the expansion of opportunity prostitution the often pursued campaign [to stop the spread of venereal diseases] was unfortunately unsuccessful."[25] Moreover, some women simply did not register as prostitutes in order to avoid supervision.[26]

In East Africa, a number of prostitutes avoided inspections through marriage, much to the consternation of public health officials. In the 1911/12 medical report, it was noted that in Iringa and in other locations marriage became "very popular in order for the women to avoid the very unpleasant control." According to German physicians, this situation contributed to the spread of VD.[27] Moreover, this interpretation undoubtedly served to reinforce the perception that many African wives were also prostitutes.

Other individuals avoided health supervision by simply leaving the area. As one physician in Cameroon reported, "an earlier attempt to put all prostitutes in Douala under police control failed as a result of the fluctuation in the population."[28] Similarly in Lomé, Togo, a colleague wrote that prostitutes simply left the region.[29] Dr. Exner in East Africa complained that when the district officer in Mohoro implemented more stringent surveillance measures for prostitutes, "those targeted quickly left" only to eventually return without being noticed.[30]

Indeed, one of the more common ways that indigenes responded to German public health methods was through movement or migration either within the colony or between different European possessions. As scholars of British and French Africa have noted, autochthons often responded to colonial policies they disliked by moving from one region to another and even from the colony of one European power to that of another.[31] Often, this migration was the result of the economic dislocations that accompanied European colonialism. At any rate, as the previously mentioned examples illustrate, Africans, Asians, and Pacific Islanders did employ migration as a means to resist health policies.

On the Marshall Islands, one medical official complained that the population there was repeatedly on the go, which made it impossible to regulate prostitution and hence the spread of venereal disease. He added that the only way to fight VD was to eliminate their freedom of movement, though this would most likely reduce the economic output of the colony. Therefore, another solution had to be found. He suggested that "the most success would likely be achieved through physician visits to the atolls and through the stationing of medical assistants to them."[32] Due to limited resources, this was an unlikely course of action.

Migration, though, may not have explicitly been used as a vehicle for noncompliance. Rather, it may have simply been a regular, preexisting pattern. For instance, in the Pacific, the migration of peoples was a common occurrence, even before the establishment of European colonies.[33] A similar situation existed in Africa, where people moved along either already existing trade routes or new ones promoted by German colonial officials.[34] Hence, traveling with trade caravans may not have constituted a conscious attempt to avoid medical control, but it nonetheless enabled some indigenes to evade it, much to the consternation of German physicians.[35]

Without a doubt, the resource issue as well as indigenous agency did explain the lack of satisfactory results for German doctors. For most physicians, however, the primary cause was non-European comportment. From their perspective, indigenes' ongoing "lax morals,"[36] "indolence,"[37] "ignorance,"[38] and even "indifference"[39] contributed significantly to the ongoing spread of VD. This indifference was also noted among the white population,[40] in particular among the lower-class elements in colonial society. One physician in DSWA complained that this indifference led to many whites not seeking treatment or receiving "improper treatment from friends or quacks." Consequently, they continued to spread the diseases through their behavior.[41]

For middle-class whites, though, German doctors attributed noncompliance to shame and not to indifference or indolence. Shame used to be prevalent in Germany until the advent of public health insurance transformed venereal infections, above all syphilis, from a moral into a medical issue.[42] However, one colonial physician believed that fear of public ridicule or shame still existed in the colonies. In the 1907/08 draft report, the local doctor in Douala remarked that "the fear of the 'self-inflected disease,' a concept which still plays a role for both civil servants and those contracted by companies (in Germany one has commendably stopped using it in the general health practice), is the main reason" many whites treat themselves.[43] Dr. Wohlgemuth noted a similar condition in DSWA: "The white bureaucrat, who was unlucky to become infected with syphilis, trustingly comes to the doctor in his district, but prefers though to go to someone who does not have an official function, and hopes to rid himself of his disease without attracting much attention."[44]

In reality, the actions of many non-Europeans and whites were most likely the result of these individuals pursuing their own agendas. For instance, for those women who engaged in prostitution, registration and the possibility of forced treatment could have caused an interruption in their source of livelihood. Therefore they utilized various strategies to get around the policies, such as citing circumstance, not registering, moving, or even marrying. Moreover, those Africans, Asians, or Pacific Islanders not accustomed to limitations on their freedom or who continued to believe in their own methods of treatment may also have adopted different strategies to avoid either detection or treatment. Thus, avoidance or withdrawal became viable options, similar to the responses they had in the precolonial period.[45]

Similarly, white private citizens and civil servants may also have avoided health surveillance for a variety of reasons. Some may have indeed felt shame and hence visited a private physician, which was not uncommon for nonmilitary whites. Meanwhile, others either sought out additional sources of treatment through alternative forms of healing, or treated themselves, or did not even seek treatment.[46] These other options may have been selected out of concerns for cost or even a lack of confidence or belief in modern Western medicine. The latter certainly applied to those seeking alternative forms of medicine in Germany.[47]

Moreover, because their status as either German citizens or foreign nationals, it was difficult to require them to undergo regular health examinations or even treatment. Admittedly, and as revealed by statistical evidence, some did go to government doctors. In DSWA, the mining company in Tsumeb attempted to induce workers to visit the company doctor by offering free treatment for those who willingly came and provided information on the source of their infection.[48] Nonetheless, the primary recipients of better health care in the overseas territories and an important source of infection in some locations remained largely outside public health control.

For autochthons, mistrust in German authorities may have contributed to their decision not to go to a German doctor. This view was even supported by colonial doctors and officials.[49] Governor Seitz in DSWA stated that though some Africans may have preferred to go to a German physician, their experiences with other German colonial institutions elicited a degree of mistrust that was difficult to overcome.[50] In East Africa, one doctor remarked that the rumors surrounding the control of prostitution led to the "unpopularity of the doctor, indeed the fear of him." He reported that this view of German physicians often resulted in the entire female population in some villages and on some plantations hiding from him before his arrival.[51] Such a perception existed in other colonies as well. According to a missionary report on DSWA, indigenes there believed that their examinations and treatments "were merely undertaken in the interest of white men."[52] One year later, an official in Windhoek said that any attempt to use force would fail. He recommended that trust needed to be established between German doctors and Africans.[53]

Other reports cited a variety of different reasons for the mistrust. Some indicated that physicians often mistreated or were unfriendly toward patients or that female patients felt extremely uncomfortable being examined by male doctors. One report from DSWA suggested health measures were often too aggressive, especially in those instances when entire communities were subjected to medical examinations against their will. In Cameroon, one physician commented that because examinations took place in a prison, many indigenes were disinclined to seek medical assistance.[54] In all these instances, the comportment of male German medical professionals and colonial authorities contributed to indigenous attitudes and behavior, which often resulted in them avoiding public health measures.

The actual methods of examination and treatment most likely also contributed to some non-Europeans and Europeans avoiding physicians or leaving treatment. Indeed, many of them often resulted in physical and even emotional discomfort for the patients. For example, the examination of indigenous women often created uncomfortable situations for the patients.[55] In contrast to men, these examinations were more invasive because often the sites of infection were not external, but rather largely internal (primarily in the cervix, though physicians at the time were not entirely certain of this). Moreover, the cures themselves could also be uncomfortable or even painful. Mercury and Salvarsan treatments were especially unpleasant experiences for patients and could even lead to death.[56] In one report out of DSWA, the local official noted that the "considerable painful symptoms during treatment and the ongoing weakening of the body for a longer time" acted as deterrents to Africans seeking an otherwise "successful treatment."[57]

These unwelcome side effects were closely connected to the limitations of medical knowledge at the time. As a matter of fact, the existence of varying courses of treatments for gonorrhea and syphilis indicated that even doctors were not confident in their overall efficacy. This was particularly evident when diseases would reappear after a course of treatment, which was common due to the absence of a true cure at the time. Most addressed the superficial symptoms of the diseases and not the bacteria that caused them. Physicians were confident that they eventually would find a cure, such as with the discovery of Salvarsan. With it and its successor, Neosalvarsan, physicians believed that they now had drugs at their disposal that promised great success in the fight against syphilis and related diseases. However, as previously mentioned, the drugs had unpleasant side effects and doctors were still uncertain about the correct dosage and means of administering the therapy. It was not until the appearance of penicillin in the 1940s that a true wonder drug was discovered.[58]

In some instances, German doctors did not even entirely comprehend the true nature of a disease. This certainly applied initially to yaws, which for years had been mistaken for syphilis. It was not until the first decade of the twentieth century that doctors were able to differentiate between the two with any regularity. The limits of medical knowledge were also apparent in the uncertainty surrounding how to treat cases of venereal granuloma.

Thus, while doctors declared many patients "cured," many probably were not. Hence, while some patients no longer carried signs of the disease, they may have still nonetheless been carriers of the disease. In some reports, most notably those for colonial soldiers, doctors used the term "ready for service" (*dienstfähig*) and noted "healed" to describe those discharged.[59] Hence, to a degree the apparent primary concern was whether or not they were capable of carrying out their functions as soldiers, not whether they were healed.

This also applied to workers. As previously stated, one of the main goals of public health policy in colonies was to ensure a steady supply of labor, both in the present and in the future. In fact, maintaining economic productivity was at times more important than the implementation of effective public health measures, as the example of migrant labor in the Marshall Islands illustrated. A similar situation existed in Southwest Africa, where the availability of workers was significantly reduced by the genocidal military policy pursued during the 1904–1907 wars against the Nama and Herero.[60] As a result of the labor shortage, the local health official in Windhoek in a memorandum argued that "it will hardly be possible to remove these people all at once from their work" for treatment, especially because "a large number" of them were "young, strong people."[61] Consequently, he stated that the ill would be identified and treated in smaller groups in order to ensure a consistent supply of labor, a decision that completely disregarded arguments that infected Africans were a major source of spreading VD.

These shortcomings of modern medicine may have prompted both non-Europeans and Europeans to seek out alternative forms of treatment. For instance, on numerous occasions doctors reported that indigenes often went to healers in their own communities: "They prefer to go in the bush, in order to have themselves treated according to their old methods, rather than to go to Windhoek, to someone who in their opinion does not offer a certain future."[62] As previously mentioned, some whites went to non–state examined individuals who practiced alternative forms of medicine.

Notes

1. For example, Levine, *Prostitution, Race and Politics,* 90.
2. Evans, "Prostitution, State and Society," 106–126; Jenders and Müller, *"Nur die Dummen,"* 39; Sauerteig, *Krankheit, Sexualität, Gesellschaft,* 68–88.
3. *MB 1908/09* (1910): 511.
4. Ibid.
5. Bethge, Bericht über die sanitären Verhältnisse vom 1.2.–31.3.13, 1 April 1913, BArch R1001/5764, 16.
6. Dr. Born, Regierungsarzt Jaluit, Medical Report, 24 June 1910, NAA G2/U24, 8.
7. *MB 1906/07* (1908): 172.
8. *MB 1905/06* (1907): 80.
9. *MB 1910/11* (1913): 586.
10. *MB 1904/05* (1906): 74.
11. *MB 1909/10* (1911): 397.
12. *MB 1908/09* (1910): 215.
13. *MB 1905/06* (1907): 392; *AkG* (1904): 53, 54; Bericht des Regierungsarztes [in Viktoria] für die Zeit vom 1 October–31 December 1906, 1906, BArch R1001/5762, 317; District Officer, Lüderitzbucht, to Imperial Government, Windhoek, 9 November 1911, BArch R151F/H.ii.h.3, 60–61.
14. Levine, *Prostitution, Race and Politics,* 70–75.
15. Petzoldt, 1. Bericht aus dem Syphilis-Krankenlager, 22 January 1914, BArch R1001/5962, 147; Petzoldt, 2. Bericht aus dem Syphilis-Krankenlager, 1 April 1914, BArch R1001/5962, 147; Petzoldt, 3. Bericht aus dem Syphilis-Krankenlager, 1 June 1914, BArch R1001/5962, 153–155.
16. Isobe, *Medizin und Kolonialismus*; Eckart, "Arzneimittelerprobung," 29–35.
17. Born, Die gesundheitliche Verhältnisse auf dem Atoll Ebon, November 1913, BArch R1001/5788: 30.
18. *AkG* (1898): 634.
19. Born, Die gesundheitliche Verhältnisse auf dem Atoll Ebon. Anhang, November 1913 BArch R1001/5788, 30.
20. Arthur Knoll, "Decision-Making for the German Colonies," in *Germans in the Tropics: Essays in German Colonial History,* ed. Knoll and Lewis Gann (New York: Greenwood Press, 1987),

131–149, 132, 144; W. O. Henderson, *Studies in German Colonial History* (Chicago: Quadrangle Books, 1962), 34; Woodruff Smith, *The German Colonial Empire* (Chapel Hill: University of North Carolina Press, 1978), 156; Horst Gründer, *Geschichte der deutschen Kolonien* (Paderborn: Ferdinand Schönigh, 1991 [1985]), 239, 242; Rudin, *Germans in the Cameroons,* 141–152.

21. Dr. Born, Medical Report, 24 June 1910, NAA G2/U24: 8; and Born, Medical Report, 4 March 1914, 61–63.
22. Eckart, *Medizin und Kolonialimperialismus,* 120–121.
23. The total area of Germany's colonies, excluding Qingdao, amounted to approximately 2,929,231 square kilometers (DSWA = 835,100 sq. km; DOA = 995,000 sq. km; Togo = 86,800 sq. km; Cameroon = 760,000 sq. km; DNG = 249,500 sq. km; and German Samoa = 2,831 sq. km), while Imperial Germany was approximately 540,857 square kilometers.
24. *AkG* (1904): 576; *MB 1907/08* (1909): 201.
25. *MB 1905/06* (1907): 199.
26. *AkG* (1902–1903): 407.
27. *MB 1911/12* (1913): 172, 171.
28. *MB 1907/08* (1909): 201.
29. *MB 1904/05* (1907): 121.
30. *MB 1911/12* (1913): 170.
31. A. I. Asiwaju, "Migration as Revolt: The examples of Ivory Coast and Upper Volta before 1945," *Journal of African History* 14 (1976): 577–594; M. C. Musambachime, "Protest Migrations in Mweru-Luapula 1900–1940," *African Studies* 47 (1988): 19–34.
32. District Officer, Jaluit, to RKA State Secretary, 24 January 1911, BArch R1001/5787, 188–189.
33. Stephen Castles, "Migrant Settlement, Transnational Communities and State Strategies in the Asia Pacific Region," in *Migration in the Asia Pacific: Population, Settlement and Citizenship Issues,* ed. Robyn Iredale, Charles Hawksley, and Stephen Castles (Northampton, MA: Edward Elgar, 2003). 3–26; B. Malinowski, "Kula: The Circulating Exchange of Valuable in the Archipelagoes of Eastern New Guinea," in *Peoples of the Pacific: The History of Oceania to 1870,* ed. Paul D'Arcy (Burlington, VT: Ashgate/Variorum, 2008), 261–270; Dorothy Shineberg, "The Sandalwood Trade in Melanesian Economics, 1841–65," in *Peoples of the Pacific,* 359–376.
34. Knoll, *Togo under Imperial Germany,* 28–30; Koponen, *Development for Exploitation,* 153, 177–183; Peter Sebald, "Togo 1884–1900," in *German Imperialism in Africa: From the Beginnings until the Second World War,* ed. Helmuth Stoecker, trans. Bernd Zollner (London: C. Hurst & Company, 1986), 89.
35. For example, see *MB 1905/06* (1907): 357; *MB1911/12* (1915), 420.
36. *AkG* (1898): 634; *MB 1905/06* (1907): 198.
37. *MB 1905/06* (1907): 359; *MB 1907/08* (1909): 77; Jäger, "Beiträge zur Rassenhygiene," 335, 334.
38. *MB 1905/06* (1907): 157; *MB 1908/09* (1910): 282.
39. *MB 1909/10* (1911): 397.
40. For example, see *AkG* (1904): 100.
41. *MB 1910/11* (1913): 587.
42. Sauerteig, "'The Fatherland is in danger,'" 76–92.
43. Jahresbericht der Stadt- und Regierungshospital in Duala 1907/08. Krankenbewegung, 1909, BArch R1001/6012, 33–34. In the final report, this sentence was missing. *MB 1907/08* (1909): 200.
44. Wohlgemuth to Imperial Government in Winhoek, 30 May 1911, BArch R151F/H.ii.H.3, 31.
45. For example, Michael Adas, "From Avoidance to Confrontation: Peasant Protest in Precolonial and Colonial Southeast Asia," *Comparative Studies in Society and History,* 23, no. 2 (1981): 217–247.

46. *MB 1910/11* (1913): 586–587.
47. Sauerteig, *Krankheit, Sexualität, Gesellschaft,* 421–423; Spree, "Kurpfuscherei," 103–121.
48. District Officer, Grootfontein, to Imperial Government, Windhoek, 10 April 1913, BArch R151F/H.ii.H.2, 9–10.
49. *AkG* (1904): 576.
50. Seitz to RKA, 24 September 1911, BArch R1001/6042, 66.
51. *MB 1911/12* (1913): 171.
52. Präses to Imperial Government in Windhoek, 11 April 1910, BArch R151F/H.ii.h.i, 75–76.
53. District Officer, Windhoek, to Imperial Goverment, Windhoek, 21 June 1911, BArch R151F/H.ii.H.3, 43.
54. Rechenberg, Runderlass an Sanitätsdienststellen und Regierungsärzte, 24 August 1911, BArch R1001/5671, 127; Conze to Dr. Petzold, 13 March 1913, BArch R1001/5962, 143–144; Seitz to RKA, 12 March 1912, BArch R1001/6010, 61–62; Dr. Hausch, Cameroon, Vorläufiger Vertieljahresbericht 1 July–30 September 1913, 1 October 1913, BArch R1001/5764, 91.
55. Conze to Dr. Petzold, 13 March 1913, 143–144; District Officer, Windhoek, to Imperial Government, Windhoek, 21 June 1911, 42.
56. Oriel, *Scar of Venus,* 81–94, 137–138, 140–145; Sauerteig, *Krankheit, Sexualität, Gesellschaft,* 34; Sauerteig, "Salvarsan und der 'ärztliche Polizeistaat,'" 166–169.
57. District Officer to Imperial Government, 21 June 1911.
58. Sauerteig, *Krankheit, Sexualität,* Gesellschaft, 34–37; Oriel, 84–94, 145, 147; Sauerteig, "Salvarsan und der 'ärztliche Polizeistaat,'" 166–169.
59. See appendix, tables 5 and 8.
60. Jürgen Zimmerer and Joachim Zeller, *Genocide in German South-West Africa: The Colonial War (1904–1908) in Namibia and its aftermath* (Monmouth, Wales: Merlin Press, 2008); Andreas Bühler, *Der Namaaufstand gegen die deutsche Kolonialherrschaft in Namibia von 1904 bis 1913* (Frankfurt: IKO, Verlag für Interkulturelle Kommunikation, 2003); Horst Drechsler, *"Let Us Die Fighting": The Struggle of the Nama and Herero against German Imperialism,* trans. Bernd Zollner (London: Zed Press, 1980); Helmut Bley, *Namibia under German Rule* (Hamburg: Lit, 1996).
61. Denkschrift zur Bekämpfung der Geschlechtskrankheiten, 5 November 1908, 20–21.
62. Wohlgemuth to Imperial Government in Winhoek, 30 May 1911.

Conclusion

Physicians in Germany and the colonies shared a desire to transform society according to their notions of health, prosperity, and morality. Within the context of the fight against venereal diseases, doctors in both settings tried to implement similar educational and surveillance measures in order to subjectify targeted groups or at least to mitigate the impact of noncompliance with prescribed measures. At times, the obstacles they faced were analogous, such as their struggle to supplant unscientific knowledge with scientifically based practices. In Germany, it was the campaign against "quackery," in the colonies it was against both the "quackery" practiced by some whites and indigenous knowledge. In other words, in the metropole and in the colonies, physicians were agents of modernity.

In both locations, doctors used similar terminology to objectify the targeted groups in order to justify the pursuit of policies aimed at bringing about their subjectification either through direct educational programs or surveillance measures. At home, physicians described their public health policies in social hygienic terms because the primary objects of the policies were members of the lower classes. Doctors classified patients as "ill" individuals, who needed to be separated from the healthy segments of society. Further, they categorized them as belonging to a group that possessed character traits threatening the social and political order, such as "ignorance," "laziness," or "indifference." This group needed to be educated and placed under surveillance.

In the colonial setting, even though the policies at their core were essentially the same as in the metropole, German physicians employed racial hygienic rhetoric because non-Europeans became the main object of the various measures they pursued. Doctors viewed Africans, Asians, and Pacific Islanders through

Notes for this section begin on page 135.

two biological lenses. First, they categorized them as "diseased" individuals when the infected appeared in the medical statistics. As in Germany, they were placed under medical surveillance and hence segregated from the healthy population until they no longer posed a threat. Second, physicians saw them as potentially dangerous because they were members of a group that exhibited traits that undermined public health policies. Doctors described non-Europeans as "lazy," "immoral," "ignorant," "indolent," and indifferent." Thus, they possessed many of the characteristics physicians ascribed to the lower classes. However, in the colonial setting they became racial attributes because they were associated with non-Europeans. Moreover, in the medical rhetoric, all non-Europeans essentially became the same regardless of their ethnicity or sex. In other words, like their lower-class counterparts in Germany, the behavior of individuals was explained via a group identity that applied essentially to Africans, Asians, and Pacific Islanders throughout the German colonial empire. This was most evident in the use of the "colored" category. Consequently, doctors saw all non-Europeans as objects needing education and surveillance.

The racial hierarchy in the colonies placed non-Europeans in a subordinate position to Europeans. Because of this status, indigenes often became the objects of medical experimentations. Hence, their position in the colonial setting was comparable to those groups in German society that were used for medical testing, such as children, prostitutes, and the mentally ill. In the context of the campaign against VD, non-Europeans became test subjects to determine the best way to administer Salvarsan and the correct dosage to use for it. The findings would later be applied to patients in Germany.

In contrast to Germany, though, the marginalized status of non-Europeans empowered German health officials to place broader segments of the Asian, African, and Pacific Islander populations under medical regulation than possible at home. German colonial physicians not only put prostitutes and military personnel under surveillance, but also those portions of the "colored" population that were either connected to the spread of VD or deemed essential to the colonial endeavor. They included laborers or those individuals under the direct control of the colonial administration, such as prisoners or government employees. In addition, because of European perceptions of non-European women, doctors assumed they were all prostitutes and therefore should be subject to medical scrutiny. Thus, German colonial authorities were able to go beyond what their colleagues were able to do in the British colonies. In the British possessions, policies targeted only military personnel and prostitutes in the context of fighting venereal diseases. Admittedly, German doctors also identified lower-class whites in the colonies as potential threats, but because of their "whiteness," they could not subject them to the same degree of surveillance as the racial "other."

More significantly, the racial hierarchy also enabled physicians to go beyond what was legally possible at home in terms of ensuring treatments were completed, which simultaneously served a didactic purpose. In some of the overseas territories, doctors increasingly resorted to various methods to guarantee that infected individuals completed their cure, especially as other methods did not achieve the desired results. Patients were more and more confined to special barracks, which at times had guards, or even prevented them from leaving treatment by erecting fences. Such facilities, though, were not used as extensively as lock hospitals were in the British colonies.[1]

In both Germany and its colonies on the eve of World War I, doctors achieved qualified success in their campaign to stop the spread of venereal diseases. While advances were made in bringing more bodies under surveillance and new treatments had been discovered, health officials still viewed VD as a threat to the economic and political order. In the overseas territories, the overall efficacy of the measures was primarily due to the behavior of the targeted populations. Though each action was primarily made by an individual, collectively they influenced the measures pursued.

Many individuals, either willingly or through surveillance tactics, did comply with the policies. For example, fathers in Cameroon often required their future sons-in-law to be free of VD before they could marry their daughters, and prostitutes needed a clean bill of health in order to earn an income. In addition, there was an increase over the years in the number of registered and cured patients, which some doctors attributed to their various normative endeavors.

However, many non-Europeans continued to behave in a manner that was seen as threatening to the political, economic, and military vitality of the colonies. In order words, Africans, Asians, and Pacific Islanders still comported themselves according to the traits Germans doctors had ascribed to them. This often led to changes in policies. For instance, in response to indigenes avoiding German doctors because of how they were treated, some German officials advocated the adoption of a friendlier attitude toward autochthons in order to convince them to seek out European medical assistance. Most changes, though, resulted in the implementation of broader and deeper surveillance measures. Physicians increasingly subjected more groups to medical supervision or limited their freedom until healed. Such measures aimed not only to limit the spread of venereal diseases in the short term by removing threats from the healthy population until cured, but also to educate them in appropriate behavior so that they would no longer pose a threat or would remove themselves willingly until treated. Such steps were justified within the context of protecting the public health of the overseas territories. So instead of focusing primarily on punitive violence and force, doctors concentrated on medical and racial discourses that aimed to discipline the colonized and ultimately legitimized those measures because targeted groups did not conform to bourgeois notions of health, work, and morality.

Consequently, this book has made more visible the less obvious ways power was exercised by colonial authorities and simultaneously revealed the limits of German rule. Though in many ways similar to efforts in the metropole, the campaign to stop the spread of VD in Germany's overseas territories was facilitated by a system based on a racial hierarchy and medical discourse that enabled medical authorities to pursue policies that ultimately enabled physicians to go beyond the scope and depth of what was possible at home. In other words, while doctors pursued a similar goal and approach in both places (education and surveillance), the frame of reference was different. In Germany, difference was based on class, while in the colonies it was predicated primarily on a concept of race closely tied to middle-class norms. This shift allowed physicians to exert a degree of surveillance impossible in Germany. In the homeland, public health measures relied primarily on the national health care system to monitor public health. And, in terms of direct control, only prostitutes and soldiers were subjected to requisite medical supervision, similar to the situation in Britain and the British colonies through the Contagious Disease Acts. Meanwhile, in the German overseas territories, supervision went beyond these two groups to include those segments of the non-European population viewed either as essential for the colonial endeavor or as threatening to it. Moreover, physicians subjected diseased bodies to greater supervision than was legally permissible at home. In Germany it would not be until the Third Reich when doctors would surpass the methods used in the colonies.

Even though they did not achieve the success they desired, through their actions colonial physicians helped buttress and justify German rule overseas. As Philippa Levine has demonstrated for parts of the British Empire, the ongoing threat of prostitution and venereal diseases necessitated the need for medical supervision, and thereby justified the continuation of colonial rule.[2] This also applied to the German situation. In the case of the struggle against VD, physicians' perceptions of indigenes and some whites revealed the necessity of continued and even increased medical control. This helped justify German rule over these populations by demonstrating the "inferiority" of non-Europeans and the "superiority" of Germans as exemplified through the possession of scientific knowledge. Further, through discourses and actions the doctors supported German colonialism by combating medical threats to it. Although they did it in the name of public health, physicians nonetheless worked to maintain the health of the cornerstones of the colonial enterprise—namely whites, soldiers, and workers—and hence supported the paradigm of male sexuality and German colonial rule.

Notes

1. Levine, *Prostitution, Race and Politics,* 70–76.
2. Ibid., 90; Levine, "'A Multitude of Unchaste Women,'" 159–163.

Appendix

Table 1. Venereal Diseases in German Togo, 1903/04 to 1911/12

"Europeans"	**1903/ 04**[1]	**1904/ 05**[2]	**1905/ 06**[3]	**1906/ 07**[4]	**1907/ 08**[5]	**1908/ 09**[6]	**1909/ 10**[7]	**1910/ 11**[8]	**1911/ 12**[9]
cases		2	86	105	80	96	127	118	85
healed		2	7	81	12	81	73	63	63
elsewhere				23		12	48		
died						1			
still in treatment				1	1	2	6		
days in hospital			94	111	32	62	142		
days in clinic				1,364	366	384	2,409		

[1]No report in *MB* for this year.

[2]Does not include information about number of days treated. Most likely incomplete based on following year's numbers.

[3]Only includes complete data for 7 patients treated in Nachtigal Hospital in Anecho.

[4]Apparently no cases in Anecho report (other diseases, but no VD), so only includes data for Lomé.

[5]Includes for first time Misahöhe. Also, data for Lomé only indicated number treated, so data incomplete.

[6]Includes Lomé, Anecho, and Palime (in Misahöhe district). No healed in Anecho, but many reported "elsewhere." In Lomé, described healed as "released," not "healed."

[7]Includes Lomé, Anecho, and Palime.

[8]Reports now only included number of cases, healed and died (and "Europeans" next to "colored" in same table) for Lomé, Anecho, and Palime.

[9]Reports now only included number of cases, healed and died (and "Europeans" next to "colored" in same table) for Lomé, Anecho, and Misahöhe.

"Coloreds"	1903/ 04[1]	1904/ 05[2]	1905/ 06[3]	1906/ 07[4]	1907/ 08[5]	1908/ 09[6]	1909/ 10[7]	1910/ 11[8]	1911/ 12[9]
cases		11	185	162	251	362	323	282	311
healed				119	89	234	205	170	240
elsewhere				36	55	117	106		
died					1	2			
still in treatment				7	12	9	12		
days in hospital				517	12	544	374		
days in clinic				2,496	3,343	1,550	6,480		

[1]No report in *MB* for this year.

[2]Only indicated the number of cases that were treated. Most likely incomplete based on follow year's numbers.

[3]Only indicated number treated.

[4]For Lomé, reported as "natives," for Anecho as "coloreds."

[5]For first time includes Misahöhe. Data for Lomé only indicated number treated and 1 died, so it is incomplete.

[6]Includes Lomé, Anecho, and Palime (in the Misahöhe district). No healed in Anecho, but many reported "elsewhere." In Lomé, described healed as "released," not "healed."

[7]Includes Lomé, Anecho, and Palime.

[8]First time "Europeans" and "colored" reported in same table, which now only included number of cases, healed and died. Data for Lomé, Anecho, Palime.

[9]"Europeans" and "colored" reported in same table, which now only included number of cases, healed and died. Data for Lomé, Anecho, and Misahöhe.

Sources: *MB 1905/06* (1907): 202, 205, 229, 231, 233; *MB 1906/07* (1908): 149, 152, 159; *MB 1907/08* (1909): 258, 273, 277, 285, 288; *MB 1908/09* (1910): 315, 320, 323, 326, 330, 332; *MB 1908/1909* (1911): 449, 454, 458, 462, 466, 468-9; *MB 1910/11* (1913): 508, 514, 518; *MB 1911/12* (1915): 459, 464, 469.

Table 2. Venereal Diseases among "European" And "Coloreds" in Togo's Main Districts, 1904/05 to 1910/11

	Lomé		Anecho		Palime/Misahöhe		Totals	
	"European"	"Colored"	"European"	"Colored"	"European"	"Colored"	"European"	"Colored"
1904/05	(no report this year)				(no report this year)			
gonorrhea			1	11			1	11
epididymitis				5				5
syphilis			1	11			1	11
Total			2	27			2	27
1905/06					(no report this year)			
gonorrhea	36	45	10	14			46	59
genital warts	1						1	0
epididymitis	2	15	2	19			4	34
ulcus molle	16	17		1			16	18
bubo	8	16	9	6			17	22
syphilis	4	26	2	26			6	52
Total	67	119	23	66			90	185
1906/07					(no report this year)			
gonorrhea	62	51		32			62	83
genital warts	3						3	0
epididymitis	2	10					2	10
ulcus molle	16	9		1			16	10
bubo	8	6					8	6
syphilis	14	41		12			14	53
Total	105	117	0	45			105	162
1907/08								
gonorrhea	41	62	8	37	2	47	51	146
genital warts	2						2	
epididymitis	2	8		1			2	9
ulcus molle	9	5		3		5	9	13
bubo	3	0		3		4	3	7
syphilis	10	20	2	34	1	22	13	76
Total	67	95	10	78	3	78	80	251
1908/09								
gonorrhea	30[1]	150[3]	5	38	8	43	43	231
genital warts	1						1	0
epididymitis	8	15		5	1		9	20
ulcus molle	11	16	1	6	1	7	13	29
bubo		0		9		6	0	15
syphilis	22[2]	29	2	28	6	10	30	67
Total	72	210	8	86	16	66	96	362
1909/10								
gonorrhea	52[4]	129[6]	12	34	8	35[7]	72	198
genital warts	5						5	0
epididymitis	4	9	1	12		2	5	23
ulcus molle	13	9	2	1	2	4[8]	17	14
bubo	4			13		3	4	16
syphilis	19[5]	15	3	49	2	8	24	72
Total	97	162	18	109	12	52	127	323

1910/11								
gonorrhea	53	94	10	32	7	22	70	148
genital warts	1						1	
epididymitis	4	24	2	7			6	31
ulcus molle	12	20		3		4	12	27
bubo	13		7	12		2	20	14
syphilis	8	20	1	35		7	9	62
Total	91	158	20	89	7	35	118	282
1911/12								
gonorrhea	46	124	4	37	4	21	54	182
genital warts	1	1	1				2	1
epididymitis	6	16		4			6	20
ulcus molle	11	26				2	11	28
bubo		4		12	2	8	2	24
syphilis	8	32		12	2	12	10	56
Total	72	203	5	65	8	43	85	311

[1]Includes 19 acute and 11 chronic cases.

[2]Includes 6 cases of stage-one syphilis, 12 cases of second stage, and 4 cases of third-stage syphilis.

[3]Includes 76 men and 74 women with gonorrhea.

[4]Includes 40 acute and 12 chronic cases.

[5]Includes 8 cases of primary, 10 cases of second-stage, and 1 case of third-stage syphilis.

[6]Includes 73 men and 56 women with gonorrhea.

[7]Includes 1 case of gonorrhic stomach-muscle abscess (Gonorrh. Bauchmuskelabzess).

[8]Includes 1 case of phagedenic chancroid.

Sources: *MB 1904/05* (1907): 126, 132–133; *MB 1905/06* (1907): 202, 205, 229, 231, 233; *MB 1906/07* (1908): 149, 152, 159; *MB 1907/08* (1909): 258, 273, 277, 285, 288; *MB 1908/09* (1910): 315, 320, 323, 326, 330, 332; *MB 1908/09* (1911): 449, 454, 458, 462, 466, 468–469; *MB 1910/11* (1913): 508, 514, 518; *MB 1911/12* (1915): 459, 464, 469.

Table 3. Venereal Diseases in German Cameroon, 1903/04 to 1911/12

"Europeans"[1]	1903/ 04[2]	1905/ 05[3]	1905/ 06[3]	1906/ 07[4]	1907/ 08[5]	1908/ 09[6]	1909/ 10	1910/ 11[7]	1911/ 12[8]
cases	7	8	6	23	52	49	44	71	154
healed	5	7	6	14	20	19	32	70	132
elsewhere		1		9	1	27	12		
died						1			
still in treatment	2				1	2			
days in hospital	117	140	134	28	230	369	472		
days in clinic				268	54	251	132		

"Coloreds"[1]	1903/ 04[2]	1904/ 05[3]	1905/ 06[4]	1906/ 07[5]	1907/ 08[5]	1908/ 09[6]	1909/ 10	1910/ 11[7]	1911/ 12[8]
cases	43	77[9]	43	211	291	392	804	1,261	1,105
healed	43	43	37	143	269	321	680	1,183	937
elsewhere		2	1	48	6	52	86		
died		1		11		4		12	3
still in treatment			5	9	16	15	38		
days in hospital	533	738	621	3,240	5,393	6,721	8,010		
days in clinic	138	321		970	3,025	1,947	9,290		

[1]Only included civilians.

[2]Included only Douala, Victoria; no reported cases for Kribi.

[3]Included only Douala; no reports for Victoria and Kribi.

[4]Included Douala, Victoria, Kribi.

[5]Included Douala, Victoria, and Kribi, though report for Kribi only indicated number of cases.

[6]First appearance of report for entire colony.

[7]First time "Europeans" and "coloreds" reported in same table, which now only included number of cases, healed and died. Also included category of Chinese, even though none there.

[8]Only included number of cases, healed and died (but now excluded Chinese category).

Sources: *MB1903/04* (1905): 133, 137–138, 150–151, 159, 166; *MB 1904/05* (1907): 95, 100, 106, 107, 114–115, 123; *MB 1905/06* (1907): 144, 147; *MB 1906/07* (1908): 102, 105, 110, 113, 121, 124; *MB 1907/08* (1909): 222, 226, 230, 234, 238, 240; *MB 1908/09* (1910): 174, 178, 181, 242, 247; *MB 1909/10* (1911): 251, 256, 259, 382, 387; *MB 1910/11* (1913): 471; *MB 1911/12* (1915): 370.

Table 4. Venereal Diseases among "Europeans" And "Colored" in Cameroon's Main Districts, 1903/04 to 1910/11

	Douala		Victoria		Kribi		Totals	
	"European"	"Colored"	"European"	"Colored"	"European"	"Colored"	"European"	"Colored"
1903/04								
gonorrhea	4	23					4	23
ulcus molle		8	1			1	1	9
bubo	1	7					1	7
syphilis	11	21				2	1	4
Total	6	40	1			3	7	43
1904/05					(No report this year)			
gonorrhea	2	13		9			2	13
epididymitis		6		1				6
ulcus molle	1	9	2	6			3	18
bubo	2			13			2	6
syphilis	3	11		21			3	13
Total	8	392	2	31			10	70
1905/06			(No report this year)		(No report this year)			
gonorrhea	4	13					4	13
ulcus molle		7						7
bubo		18						18
syphilis	2	5					2	5
Total	6	43					6	43
1906/07								
gonorrhea	3	45	1	15	5	38	9	98
genital warts		1						1
epididymitis	1	1			1	12	2	13
ulcus molle	1	12	1	4		6	2	22
bubo	1	13		5	1	31	2	49
syphilis	5	10		8	3	10	8	28
Total	11	82	2	32	10	97	23	211
1907/08								
gonorrhea	2	39	9	81	12	11	23	131
genital warts		1		1				2
epididymitis	1	1		2	1	2	2	6
ulcus molle	4	8		7	7		11	17
bubo	1	17		9	3	1	4	27
syphilis	2	52	3	55	7	1	12	108
Total	10	118	12	158	30	15	52	291
1908/093								
gonorrhea	1	45	2	27	11	1	13 (+5)	180
genital warts								(+3)
epididymitis		2		1				3 (+11)
ulcus molle	1	7		1			1	8 (+23)
bubo	2	22	1	8	3	2	6	32 (+27)
syphilis	8	21	1	18	8	1	17 (+7)	40 (+65)
Total	12	97	4	55	22	4	49	392

1909/10[3]								
gonorrhea	12	38	1	21		13	13 (+11)	72 (+374)
genital warts								(+2)
epididymitis		6				1		7 (+15)
ulcus molle		3		1		3		7 (+68)
bubo	4	15		9		7	4 (+1)	31 (+53)
syphilis	7	21	2	9	2	6	9 (+6)	26 (+149)
Total	23	83	3	40	2	30	44	804
1910/11[4]								
gonorrhea							27	649
genital warts							1	2
epididymitis							2	20
ulcus molle							5	96
bubo							18	93
syphilis							18	401
Total							71	1,261
1911/12[4]								
gonorrhea							38	543
genital warts								1
epididymitis							2	15
ulcus molle							11	129
bubo							84	98
syphilis							69	319
Total							154	1,105

[1]Tertiary syphilis.

[2]Although the report says that there were 46 new cases, some of these included patients who suffered from more than one venereal disease, such as a syphilitic individual who also suffered from gonorrhea and ulcus molle.

[3]This year the report also included for the first time statistics for the entire colony and not just the three main districts. Hence, the final two columns also include figures from other parts of the territory (the numbers in parentheses).

[4]For this year, only statistics for the entire colony presented in *MB*.

Sources: *MB1903/04* (1905): 133, 137–138, 150–151, 159, 166; *MB 1904/05* (1907): 95, 100, 106, 107, 1123, 114–115; *MB 1905/06* (1907): 144, 147; *MB 1906/07* (1908): 102, 105, 110, 113, 121, 124 ; *MB 1907/08* (1909): 222, 226, 230, 234, 238, 240; *MB 1908/09* (1910): 174, 178, 181, 242, 247; *MB 1909/1910* (1911): 251, 256, 259, 382, 387; *MB 1910/11* (1913): 471; *MB 1911/12* (1915): 370.

Table 5. Venereal Diseases among Colonial Soldiers in German Cameroon, 1900/01 to 1911/12

German Soldiers	1900/01	1901/02	1902/03	1903/04	1904/05	1905/06	1906/07	1907/08	1908/09	1909/10[3]	1910/11	1911/12
troop strength		85	71			85					114[4]	118[4]
cases		0[2]	0	0	0	2	2	4	6	0		
% of strength												
healed[1]												
sent home												
elsewhere												
died												
still												
days treated						86		25				

[1]Used the term "ready for duty" (*dienstfähig*), and not "healed"
[2]The reporting physician was surprised by this due to the high rate of infection among other sections of the population; *MB 1905/06* (1907): 389.
[3]Only a half-year report.
[4]Average, not exact number.

African Soldiers	1900/01	1901/02	1902/03	1903/04	1904/05	1905/06	1906/07	1907/08	1908/09	1909/10[2]	1910/11	1911/12
troop strength											1225[3]	1378[3]
new cases[1]	419	425	314	238	210	279	367	333	260	163	0[4]	0[5]
% of strength	42.90%	41.30%	34.50%	22.30%	21.50%	19.30%	31%	25.30%				
healed												
sent home												
elsewhere												
died												
still												
days treated						6104				4830		
% of new cases						13.40%						

[1]Does not include cases carried over from previous year.
[2]Only half-year report (October 1909–March 1910).
[3]Average, not exact number.
[4]According to report, "venereal diseases were represented the most," but no numbers were provided; *MB 1910/11* (1913): 765.
[5]According to the report, VD was "endemic" along with malaria and intestinal diseases, though no statistical evidence was provided; *MB 1911/12* (1915): 639.

Sources: *AkG* (1904): 73; *MB 1905/06* (1907): 122–123, 389, 391, 404–405, 410, 417, 419, 423, 431, 437, 438; *MB 1906/07* (1908): 314, 320, 323; *MB 1907/08* (1909): 521–522; *MB 1908/09* (1910): 503, 507, 510–511; *MB 1909/10* (1911): 629, 635, 637, 639; *MB 1910/11* (1913): 764–765; *MB 1911/12* (1915): 638, 639.

Table 6. Venereal Diseases in German Southwest Africa, 1903/04 to 1911/12

"Europeans"	1902/03[1]	1903/04[2]	1904/05[2]	1905/06[2]	1906/07[1]	1907/08[3]	1908/09[3]	1909/10[2]	1910/11[4]	1911/12[2]
cases	104				69	256	336		384	
healed						208	292		351	
elsewhere						30	35			
died						1			1	
still in treatment						17	9			
days in hospital						3,978	5,409			
days in clinic										

[1]Only included number of cases (doesn't include Schutztruppe).
[2]No publicly published report.
[3]Only includes white civilians.
[4]For this year only included data on number of cases treated (and type), healed, and died.

"Coloreds"	1902/03[1]	1903/04[2]	1904/05[2]	1905/06[2]	1906/07[3]	1907/08[4]	1908/09	1909/10[2]	1910/11[5]	1911/12[2]
cases	408				360	470	463		700	
healed						322	342		351	
elsewhere						27	73			
died						2	4		13	
still in treatment						119	44			
days in hospital						13,168	13,570			
days in clinic										

[1]Only included number of cases.
[2]No publicly published report for these years.
[3]No table, but rather narrative and refers to them as "natives." Also, apparently does not include those "natives" in prison camps.
[4]Only includes "free coloreds" and total number of days treated (not broken down btw clinic and hospital).
[5]For this year only included data on number of cases treated (and type), healed, and died.

Sources: *AkG* (1904): 596; *MB 1906/07* (1908): 172; *MB 1907/08* (1909): 316, 318, 320, 322; *MB 1908/09* (1910): 345, 347, 350, 351; *MB 1910/11* (1913): 604, 608.

Table 7. Specific Venereal Diseases in German Southwest Africa, 1907/08, 1908/09, and 1910/11

1907/08	German Soldiers	White Civilians	Africans
gonorrhea	531	80	297
genital Warts	16	5	3
epididymitis	14	23	11
ulcus molle	72	38	10
bubo	8	13	
syphilis	117	97	149
Total	758	256	470

1908/09	German Soldiers	White Civilians	Africans
gonorrhea		174	221[2]
genital Warts		1	2
epididymitis		7	8
ulcus molle		14	3
bubo		3	
syphilis		129	118
Total		328 (+8)[1]	352 (+111)[1]

1910/11	German Soldiers	White Civilians	Africans
gonorrhea		137	229
genital Warts		8	14
epididymitis		25	25
ulcus molle		5	19
bubo		8	14
syphilis		201	399
Total		384	700

[1]Figure in parentheses indicates cases not assigned to a specific disease but were still included in the report.

[2]Includes 2 also infected with ulcus molle and 2 also infected with syphilis.

Sources: *MB 1907/08* (1909): 311, 316, 320; *MB 1908/09* (1910): 345, 350; *MB 1910/11* (1913): 604.

Table 8. Venereal Diseases among German Colonial Soldiers in German Southwest Africa, 1898/99 to 1911/12

German Soldiers	1898/ 99	1899/ 00[1]	1900/ 00[1,2]	1900/ 01[1]	1901/ 02	1902/ 03[2]	1903/ 04[2]	1904/ 05[2]	1905/ 06[2]	1906/ 07[2]	1907/ 08[3]	1908/ 09	1909/ 10	1910/ 11
troop strength											6,749– 3,799			1972.86[4]
new cases	150	175	82	148	162						760			
old cases	10	18	17	20	9									
% of strength											13.83%	12.29%	8.30%	7.20%
healed		176	78	155[5]	164[5]						490[5]			
sent home											165			
elsewhere			1	1							33			
died											1			
still in treatment		16	20	9	7						71		54	
days treated	76[6]	[7]	[7]	[7]	[7]						19,440			

[1]Figures for this year do not add up correctly.

[2]No report found for this year, perhaps due to Herero and Nama Wars.

[3]Only year in which a full table was included.

[4]Average troop strength.

[5]This year described as "ready for service" (*dienstfähig) and* not as healed.

[6]Average number of treatment days.

[7]Either used average days treated or total days treated for individual diseases, but in same report. Therefore impossible to calculate data for each year.

Sources: *AkG* (1902–1903): 415, 423, 431; *AkG* (1904): 94–95, 104; *MB 1907/08* (1909): 311, 313; *MB 1910/11* (1913): 795.

Table 9. Venereal Diseases in German East Africa, 1903/04 to 1911/12

"Europeans"	**1903/04**	**1904/05**	**1905/06**	**1906/07**	**1907/08**	**1908/09**	**1909/10**	**1910/11**	**1911/12**
cases	79	84	143	140	207	232	265	302	276
healed	52	63	124	115	148	147	188	187	207
elsewhere	19	18	18	19	48	82	63		
died	1					1			
still in treatment	7	3	1	6	11	2	14		
days in hospital	340	142	749	677	541	690	838		
days in clinic	1,245	1,868	2,195	2,878	3,755	3,971	4,489		
"Coloreds"	**1903/04**	**1904/05**	**1905/06**	**1906/07**	**1907/08**	**1908/09**	**1909/10**	**1910/11**	**1911/12**
cases	996	1,053	1,029	1,188	1,708	2,000	2,012	2,144	2,650
healed	823	881	848	1,009	1,439	1,690	1,717	1,830	2,355
elsewhere	105	125	143	90	146	189	163		
died	4	9	5	5	13	15	12	7	19
still in treatment	64	38	33	84	110	106	120		
days in hospital	17,399	16,554	9,746	15,858	24,632	25,477	20,237		
days in clinic	7,774	8,883	11,514	9,126	18,565	22,162	23,802		

Sources: *MB 1903/04* (1905): 114, 120; *MB 1904/05* (1907): 68, 74; *MB 1905/06* (1907): 100, 107; *MB 1906/07* (1908): 73, 79; *MB 1907/08* (1909): 125–126, 132; *MB 1908/09* (1910): 150, 157; *MB 1909/10* (1911): 217, 224; *MB 1910/11* (1913): 355; *MB 1911/12* (1915): 238.

Table 10. Specific Venereal Diseases in German East Africa, 1903/04 to 1911/12

	1903/04		1904/05		1905/06		1906/07		1907/08		1908/09		1909/10		1910/11		1911/12	
	"Europeans"	"Coloreds"	"Europeans"	"Coloreds"	"Europeans"	"Coloreds"	"Europeans"	"Coloreds"	"Europeans"	"Coloreds"	"Europeans"	"Coloreds"	"Europeans"	"Coloreds"	"Europeans	"Coloreds"	"Europeans"	"Coloreds"
gonorrhea	3	495	36	486	55	402	55	520	97	713	111	778	123	724	145	758	136	1,016
genital warts	1	7	0	14	0	1	0	3	1	2	2	3	6	4	1	8	3	3
epididymitis	1	53	3	53	6	54	6	73	14	129	7	119	8	154	11	184	11	148
ulcus molle	12	180	12	217	26	208	30	204	32	264	35	269	41	237	42	232	29	213
bubo	8	26	7	42	13	51	10	77	18	84	23	117	14	104	18	81	17	50
syphilis	26	235	26	241	43	313	39	311	43	516	54	714	73	789	85	881	80	1,220
Total	79	996	84	1,053	143	1,029	140	1,118	207	1,708	232	2,000	265	2,012	302	2,144	276	2,650

Sources: *MB 1903/04* (1905): 114, 120; *MB 1904/05* (1907): 68, 74; *MB 1905/06* (1907): 100, 107; *MB 1906/07* (1908): 73, 79; *MB 1907/08* (1909): 125–126, 132; *MB 1908/09* (1910): 150, 157; *MB 1909/10* (1911): 217, 224; *MB 1910/11* (1913): 355; *MB 1911/12* (1915): 238.

Table 11. Venereal Diseases in Dar es Salaam, 1903/04 to 1911/12

	1903/04[1]		1904/05[1]		1905/06[1]		1906/07		1907/08		1908/09[4]		1909/10[4]		1910/11[5]		1911/12[5]	
	"Euro-peans"	"Coloreds"	"Euro-peans"	"Coloreds"	"Euro-peans"[2]	"Coloreds"	"Euro-peans"[2]	"Coloreds"	"Euro-peans"[3]	"Coloreds"	"Euro-peans"	"Coloreds"	"Euro-peans"	"Coloreds"	"Euro-peans"	"Coloreds"	"Euro-peans"	"Coloreds"
gonorrhea	5	173	3	128	24	123	22	134	39 (+7)	155					62	5	70	5
genital warts		5		10		1		3	1									
epididymitis		7		9	3	9	4	12	8	9					3		2	
ulcus molle	3	6	1	103	20	89	14	73	6 (+1)	61					26	2	8	
bubo		2	3	4	8	10	8	15	2	4					7		4	
syphilis	6	39	1	23	26	29	19	28	15 (+1)	49					44	2		
Total	14	232	8	277	81	261	67	265	71 (+9)	278					142	9		

[1]Includes government hospital in Dar es Salaam and Sewa-Hadji-Hospital for "coloreds," which included Africans, Arabs, and Asians.

[2]Records indicated that for all illnesses treated in the government hospital this year, a small number of the patients were Indian. However, there was no indication that any of them were treated for STDs.

[3]Even though the government hospital treated Indians for various illnesses, the data includes exclusively Europeans. The numbers in parentheses indicate the number of Asians treated.

[4]No data provided this year in the published report.

[5]Includes only "European" and "colored" patients treated in the government hospital, and hence excludes those treated in the exclusively non-European Sewa-Hadji-Hospital.

Sources: *MB 1903/04* (1905): 4, 11; *MB 1904/05* (1907): 4, 10; *MB 1905/06* (1907): 6, 15; *MB 1906/07* (1908): 5, 15; *MB 1907/08* (1909): 5, 8, 19-20; *MB 1910/11* (1913): 372; *MB 1911/12* (1915): 248.

Table 12. Venereal Diseases among German Colonial Soldiers in German East Africa, 1894/95 to 1911/12

German Soldiers	**1894/ 95**	**1895/ 96**	**1896/ 97**	**1897/ 98**	**1898/ 99**	**1899/ 1900**	**1900/ 01**	**1901/ 02**	**1902/ 03**	**1903/ 04**	**1904/ 05**	**1905/ 06**	**1906/ 07**	**1907/ 08**	**1908/ 09**	**1909/ 10[3]**	**1910/ 11**	**1911/ 12**
troop strength									162	130.5[2]	137.9[2]	241.8[2]	189[2]	190.8[2]	217.1[2]	204.2[2]	203[2]	228[2]
cases	14	15	17	6 new		8 new				6	9	8	11	3				
% of strength										4.60%	6.50%	3.60%	5.70%	1.50%				
healed			14															
sent home																		
elsewhere			1[1]															
died																		
still in treatment			2															
days treated																		

[1]Sent to another station. [2]Average, not exact number. [3]Only a half-year report.

African Soldiers	**1894/ 95**	**1895/ 96**	**1896/ 97**	**1897/ 98**	**1898/ 99**	**1899/ 1900**	**1900/ 01**	**1901/ 02**	**1902/ 03**	**1903/ 04**	**1904/ 05**	**1905/ 06**	**1906/ 07**	**1907/ 08**	**1908/ 09**	**1909/ 10[4]**	**1910/ 11**	**1911/ 12**
troop strength									1,805.9[3]	1,786.9[3]	1,913.7[3]	3,840.1[3]	2,691.8[3]	2,838.1[3]	2,755.1[3]	2,788.2[3]	3,065[3]	3,055[3]
cases	400	360	452	416 new		461			817[2]	740	655	744	778	770	696	339	951	853
% of strength										41.00%	39.00%	19.40%	28%	27.10%	25.20%			
healed			423			433												
sent home																		
elsewhere			11[1]															
died						2												
still in treatment			18			14												
days treated																		
% of new cases										32.50%	24.70%	13.40%	23.40%	20.10%	23.30%	18.10%	22%	17.38%

[1]Released home ("*in die Heimat*"). [3]Average number, not exact.

[2]Only included gonorrhea, syphilis, and ulcus molle. [4]Only a half-year report.

Sources: *AkG* (1897): 33; *AkG* (1898): 634; *AkG* (1899): 333; *AkG* (1899): 353; *AkG* (1902-03): 378; *MB 1905/06* (1907): 345, 355, 356, 370; *MB 1906/07* (1908): 298; *MB 1908/09* (1910): 483, 485; *MB 1909/10* (1911): 605, 607, 621; *MB 1910/11* (1913): 754; *MB 1911/12* (1915): 627, 628.

Table 13. Venereal Diseases in German New Guinea, 1897/98, 1901/02 to 1911/12

Old Protectorate "Europeans"	1903/04[1]	1904/05[2]	1905/06[3]	1906/07[4]	1907/08[4]	1908/09[5]	1909/10[6]	1910/11[7]	1911/12[8]
cases	13	12	12	15	9	27	17	31	43
healed	10		9	12	4	22	13	28	37[9]
elsewhere			1		1	3	4	3	
died									
still in treatment			2		1	2			
days in hospital	38	180	142	25	70	47	33	130	
days in clinic								150	

[1]Included Herbertshöhe and Friedrich Wilhelmshafen. Data incomplete because only included total number of treatment days for Friedrich-Wilhelmshafen without reference to hospital or clinic. Plus, for FWH no information on outcome of treatment.

[2]Included Herbertshöhe and Kaiser-Wilhelmsland. Data incomplete for outcome and days treated.

[3]Only included Herbertshöhe.

[4]Included only Herbertshöhe and Kaiser-Wilhelmsland (but data for latter only number ill and days treated).

[5]Included Herbertshöhe and Rabaul (Simpsonshafen). Data on treatment days missing for Rabaul. For Herbertshöhe did not indicate whether clinic or hospital.

[6]Includes Herbertshöhe, Rabaul, and Friedrich-Wilhelmshafen (though no reported cases for latter). Also, treatment days in Rabaul not provided for Europeans.

[7]Included Herbertshöhe, Rabaul, Friedrich-Wilhelmshafen and Käwieng. Rabaul did not report the number of treatment days.

[8]First appearance of comprehensive report (which included Rabaul, Herbertshöhe, Käwieng, South New Mecklenburg, and Friedrich-Wilhelmshafen). Compared to individual reports, this comprehensive report short one patient.

[9]In overview report, category "healed or released elsewhere."

"Coloreds"	1903/04[1]	1904/05[2]	1905/06[3]	1906/07[4]	1907/08[5]	1908/09[6,7]	1909/10[8]	1910/11[9]	1911/12[10,11]
cases	67	95	113	154	113	202	256	214	362 (+18)
healed	13		82	54	108	123	176	192	335 (+18)[12]
elsewhere			6	1	1		1	2	
died	1			1	1	1		2	
still in treatment			25	7	3	4	24	18	
days in hospital	2,988	3,903	2,146	2,078	3,189	5,405	9,189	1,116	
days in clinic			5,544					5,728	

[1]Only included Herbertshöhe and Friedrich-Wilhelmshafen (incomplete data).

[2]Only included Herbertshöhe and Kaiser-Wilhelmsland. Days treated only included Kaiser-Wilhelmsland.

[3]Included only Herbertshöhe and Käwieng.

[4]Only included Herbertshöhe and Käwieng, but data for latter only included number treated.

[5]Included only Herbertshöhe and Käwieng.

[6]Includes Herbertshöhe, Rabaul (Simpsonshafen), Kaiser-Wilhelmsland, and Käwieng. Not all data regarding what happened to patients provided or days treated.

[7]For Kaiser-Wilhelmsland also included Chinese under "Farbige."

[8]Included Herbertshöhe, Rabaul, Käwieng, and Friedrich-Wilhelmshafen (data on outcome for FWH incomplete). Moreover, data from FWH included 5 Chinese.

[9]Includes Herbertshöhe, Rabaul, and Friedrich-Wilhelmshafen.

[10]First appearance of comprehensive report (which included Rabaul, Herbertshöhe, Käwieng, South New Mecklenburg, and Friedrich-Wilhelmshafen). Compared to individual reports, this comprehensive report short one patient.

[11]Also included 18 Chinese and "nonindigenous natives" (the number in parentheses).

[12]In overview report, category "healed or released elsewhere."

Sources: *MB 1903/04* (1905): 200, 204, 230, 257; *MB 1904/05* (1907): 141, 143, 163, 171–172, 177, 180–181; *MB 1905/06* (1907): 272, 276, 298; *MB 1906/07* (1908): 216, 222, 226, 227; *MB 1907/08* (1909): 435, 440, 443, 450; *MB 1908/09* (1910): 358, 362, 378, 380, 407; *MB 1909/10* (1911): 508, 512, 515, 518, 521, 523; *MB 1910/11* (1913): 662, 665, 670, 675, 681, 684, 688; *MB 1911/12* (1915): 529, 539, 546, 550, 555, 559.

Table 14. Specific Venereal Diseases in German New Guinea Old Protectorate Districts, 1903/04 to 1911/12

	Herbertshöhe		Friedrich-Wilhelmshafen		Kaiser-Wilhelmsland		Käwieng		Rabaul		South New Mecklenburg		Total	
	"European"	"Colored"	"European"	"Colored"	"European"	"Colored"	"European"	"Colored"	"European"	"Colored"	"European"	"Colored"	"European"	"Colored"
1903/04														
gonorrhea	7	5		26									7	31
epididymitis		1												1
ulcus molle	1	6												6
syphilis	1	1		4									1	5
venereal granulum		1		10									1	11
other				13[2]										13
Total	9	14	4[1]	53									13[1]	67
1904/05														
gonorrhea	2	13			1	13							3	26
genital warts														
epididymitis					1								1	
ulcus molle		8			1								1	8
bubo														
syphilis	5	3			2	13							5	16
venereal granulum						14								14
other						31[3]								31
Total	7	24			5								12	95
1905/06														
gonorrhea	7	28						40					7	68
genital warts		4												4
epididymitis	1												1	
ulcus molle		27												27
bubo	2	5											2	5
syphilis	2	7						2					2	9
Total	12	71						42					12	113

1906/07														
gonorrhea	6	18											6	18
genital warts	1	2											1	2
epididymitis	3	3											3	3
ulcus molle		26												26
bubo	1	5											1	5
syphilis	1	4											1	4
venereal granulum		5												5
Total	12	63			3[1]	91[1]							15[1]	154[1]
1907/08														
gonorrhea	1	13						34					1	47
genital warts		7												7
epididymitis	3												3	
ulcus molle		12												12
bubo		5												5
syphilis	2	1						9						10
venereal granulum		4											2	4
other								28						28
Total	6	42			3[1]			71					9[1]	113
1908/09														
gonorrhea	7	13						31	6	18			13	62
genital warts		1						2		1				4
epididymitis	8	6											8	6
ulcus molle		11						4	4	9			4	24
bubo								6						6
syphilis		1						9	2	10			2	20
venereal granulum		4												4
other								3						3
Total	15	36				73[1]		55[4]	12	38			27	202[1]

1909/10														
gonorrhea	2	3						11	7	56			9	70
genital warts		1						2		16				19
epididymitis	1	1											1	1
ulcus molle	1	6						2		42			1	50
bubo		2								11				13
syphilis	3	2						31		2			3	35
venereal granulum		1							3	12			3	13
Total	7	16		55[1,5]				46	10	139			17	256[1]
1910/11														
gonorrhea	6	3	6	15			4		8	78			24	96
genital warts		1		4						49				54
epididymitis									1	6			1	6
ulcus molle									1	27			1	27
bubo										8				8
syphilis	1	1		4					4				5	5
venereal granulum				3						12				15
Total	7	5	6	26			4		14	180			31	211
1911/12														
gonorrhea	5	2	9	29 (+1)[8]			3	68 (+1)[8]	7	63 (+15)[9]		6	24	168 (+17)[8,9]
genital warts				7				5	2	13		1	2	26
epididymitis		5	1	3			1	4	2	32		1	4	45
ulcus molle		1					1	27	1	22			2	50
bubo								14 (+1)[8]	3	7		1	3	22 (+1)[8]
syphilis	2		1				2	13	3	1			8	14
venereal granulum				3				10		14		9		36
other		2[6]	1[7]										1	2
Total	7	10	12	42 (+1)[8]			7	141 (+2)[8]	18	152 (+15)[9]		18	44	363 (+18)[8,9]

[1]Not categorized in the report or includes uncategorized cases.

[2]All cases of ulcers on the genital phimosis.

[3]Included herpes, balanorrhoea, and other less common diseases or those that did not always allow for an accurate diagnosis; *MB 1904/05* (1907): 172.

[4]Included 6 Chinese, 2 Malayans, and 65 Melanesians.

[5]Included 5 Chinese, 4 Malayans, and 46 Melanesians.

[6]Included one case of balanorrhoea and one of phagedenic chancroid.

[7]Included one case with a prostatic abscess.

[8]The number in parentheses indicated additional patients who were Chinese.

[9]The number in parentheses included Chinese and "nonindigenous natives."

Sources: *MB 1903/04* (1905): 200, 204, 230, 257; *MB 1904/05* (1907): 141, 143, 163, 171–172, 177, 180–181; *MB 1905/06* (1907): 272, 276, 298; *MB 1906/07* (1908): 216, 222, 226, 227; *MB 1907/08* (1909): 435, 440, 443, 450; *MB 1908/09* (1910): 358, 362, 378, 380, 407; *MB 1909/10* (1911): 508, 512, 515, 518, 521, 523; *MB 1910/11* (1913): 662, 665, 670, 675, 681, 684, 688; *MB 1911/12* (1915): 529, 539, 546, 550, 555, 559.

Table 15. Specific Venereal Diseases in the Island Territories of German New Guinea, 1897/98, 1901/02 to 1911/12

	West Carolines		East Carolines		Marshall Islands			Mariana Islands		Palau Islands			Total		
	"European"	"Colored"	"European"	"Colored"	"European"	"Colored"	Chinese	"European"	"Colored"	"European"	"Colored"	Chinese	"European"	"Colored"	Chinese
1897/98															
gonorrhea															
genital warts															
epididymitis															
ulcus molle															
bubo															
syphilis						175								175	
other															
Total						175								175	
1901/02															
gonorrhea				45		17								62	
genital warts															
epididymitis															
ulcus molle				2		5								7	
bubo															
syphilis						76								76	
other															
Total				47		98								145	
1902/03															
gonorrhea				24										24	
genital warts															
epididymitis															
ulcus molle				2										2	
bubo															
syphilis															
other															
Total				26										26	

1903/04												
gonorrhea		2										2
genital warts												
epididymitis												
ulcus molle	2										2	
bubo												
syphilis		41[1]										41
other												
Total	2	43									2	43
1904/05												
gonorrhea	2	8		12							2	20
genital warts												
epididymitis		1										1
ulcus molle		2										2
bubo	1	1									1	1
syphilis		133		2								135
other												
Total	3	112		14[2]							3	159
1905/06												
gonorrhea			1	13							1	13
genital warts												
epididymitis												
ulcus molle												
bubo												
syphilis		8		6								14
Total		8	1	19							1	27
1906/07												
gonorrhea				7	2	5					2	12
genital warts												
epididymitis				4	1	4					1	8
ulcus molle						1						1
bubo						1						1
syphilis				17	3	15					3	32
Total				28	6	26					6	54

1907/08													
gonorrhea		7	1	20	5	5	2			6	32	2
genital warts							1					1
epididymitis		1				10	3				11	3
ulcus molle					2	2	1			2	2	1
bubo						1	5				1	5
syphilis		2		23	1	20	1			1	45	1
other												
Total		10	1	43	8	38	13			9	91	13
1908/09												
gonorrhea	2	11	1	4	16	27				19	42	
genital warts						1					1	
epididymitis						13					13	
ulcus molle	1	2		2	1	3				2	7	
bubo						1					1	
syphilis		1				23					24	
other			1[3]							1		
Total	3	14	2	6	17	68[4]				22	88	
1909/10												
gonorrhea	3	7	2	13	13	30		12		18	62	
genital warts						1					1	
epididymitis						4		1			5	
ulcus molle	1				1	7				2	7	
bubo						1		1			2	
syphilis		3		35	5	66		67		5	171	
other				1[5]							1	
Total	4	10	2	49	19	109[4]		81		25	249	

1910/11														
gonorrhea	1	9		10					1	3	1	2	22	1
genital warts		1											1	
epididymitis		1								2			3	
ulcus molle		4		1									5	
bubo		1											1	
syphilis		15								15			30	
other														
Total	1	31		11					1	20	1	2	62	1
1911/12														
gonorrhea	10	9	8	11	9	33			3	15	2	30	68	2
genital warts														
epididymitis		2		28	1	14						1	44	
ulcus molle		1			5	11						5	12	
bubo					3	3				8		3	11	
syphilis		11		91	3	105				14		3	221	
other				1[6]									1	
Total	10	23	8	131	21	166[4]			3	37	2	42	357	2

[1]Described as "syphilitic ulcers."

[2]For the September 1904–March 1905 reporting year.

[3]One case of "strictures of the urethra."

[4]No separate report for Chinese this year, so unclear if present or included under "colored."

[5]A case of "ulcus glandis" or "ulcerated penis."

[6]One case of "injured testicle."

Sources: *AkG* (1899): 364; *AkG* (1904): 113, 138, 614; *MB 1903/04* (1905): 274, 275 ; *MB 1904/05* (1907): 234–235, 242, 246; *MB 1905/06* (1907): 305, 307, 308; *MB 1906/07* (1908): 251, 254; *MB 1907/08* (1909): 463, 468, 471, 478, 480, 488, 491, 494, 496; *MB 1908/09* (1910): 430, 433, 436, 438, 448, 450, 456, 461; *MB 1909/10* (1911): 531, 533, 536, 537, 542, 544, 550, 554, 570; *MB 1910/11* (1913): 698, 701, 725; *MB 1911/12* (1915): 578, 592, 601, 606.

Table 16. Venereal Diseases in German Samoa, 1903/04 to 1911/12

"Europeans"	**1903/ 04**[1]	**1904/ 05**	**1905/ 06**	**1906/ 07**	**1907/ 08**	**1908/ 09**[1]	**1909/ 10**	**1910/ 11**	**1911/ 12**
cases	0	3	4	5	26	0	7	4	4
healed			2	1	16		1	4	4
elsewhere			2	4	9		5		
died									
still in treatment					1		1		
days in hospital			23				18		
days in clinic			21	29	529		24		

[1]None reported.

"Coloreds"	**1903/ 04**[1]	**1904/ 05**[2]	**1905/ 06**[3]	**1906/ 07**[4]	**1907/ 08**[5]	**1908/ 09**	**1909/ 10**	**1910/ 11**	**1911/ 12**
cases	6	13	41	67	0	72	155	68	36
healed			34	54		15	5	68	36
elsewhere			3	10		37	136		
died									
still in treatment			4	3		20	14		
days in hospital			248	607		31	40		
days in clinic			382	510		163	501		

[1]Referred to as "Samoan" and only provided information on the number of infections reported.

[2]Referred to as "Polynesian" and only included the number of cases treated in the Apia government hospital. There was a category for Melanesians, but no reported cases.

[3]First time referred to as "colored" in the comprehensive report. Appears "Chinese" included in this category this year. See *MB 1905/06* (1907): 320.

[4]No separate category for "Chinese," so like last year probably included here.

[5]None reported for this year.

Chinese	**1903/ 04**	**1904/ 05**	**1905/ 06**[1]	**1906/ 07**[1]	**1907/ 08**	**1908/ 09**	**1909/ 10**	**1910/ 11**	**1911/ 12**
cases	6	3			11	18	24	8	15
healed					9	8	7	8	15
elsewhere					2	10	14		
died									
still in treatment							3		
days in hospital					123	70	72		
days in clinic					75	137	44		

[1]Included in "colored" section this year.

Sources: *MB 1903/04* (1905): 299; *MB 1904/05* (1907): 263; *MB 1905/06* (1907): 324, 327; *MB 1906/07* (1908): 282, 286; *MB 1907/08* (1909): 506, 513; *MB 1908/09* (1910): 472, 475; *MB 1909/10* (1911): 586, 590, 593; *MB 1910/11* (1913): 742; *MB 1911/12* (1915): 616.

Table 17. Specific Venereal Diseases in German Samoa, 1903/04 to 1911/12

"Europeans"	1903/ 04[1]	1904/ 05	1905/ 06	1906/ 07	1907/ 08	1908/ 09	1909/ 10	1910/ 11	1911/ 12
gonorrhea				3	12		1		
genital warts									
epididymitis			2		4				3
ulcus molle									
bubo		1	1				2		
syphilis		1	1	2	10		4	4	1
Total	0[1]	3[2]	4	5	26	0[1]	7	4	4

[1]No reported cases.

[2]Also included a case of herpes.

"Coloreds"	1903/ 04[1]	1904/ 05[2]	1905/ 06[3]	1906/ 07[4]	1907/ 08[5]	1908/ 09	1909/ 10	1910/ 11	1911/ 12
gonorrhea	6	1	11	16		5	5	4	3
genital warts									
epididymitis			20	11		6	4		1
ulcus molle				2					1
bubo		1	3	6		2	2	5	4
syphilis		10	7	32		59	144	59	27
Total	6[6]	13[7]	41	67	0	72	155	68	36

[1]Referred to as "Samoan" and only provided information on the number of infections reported.

[2]Referred to as "Polynesian" and only included the number of cases treated in the Apia government hospital. There was a category for Melanesians, but no reported cases.

[3]First time referred to as "colored" in the comprehensive report. Appears "Chinese" included in this category this year. See *MB 1905/06* (1907): 320.

[4]No separate category for "Chinese," so like last year probably included here.

[5]No cases reported this year.

[6]Only reported total number of venereal diseases without indicating specific types.

[7]Also included a case of herpes.

Chinese	1903/ 04	1904/ 05	1905/ 06[3]	1906/ 07[3]	1907/ 08	1908/ 09	1909/ 10	1910/ 11	1911/ 12
gonorrhea					5	6	5	1	5
genital warts									1
epididymitis					5	6	5	5	6
ulcus molle						1			1
bubo						2	10	2	1
syphilis		2			1	3	4		1
Total	6[1]	3[2]			11	18	24	8	15

[1]Only reported total number of venereal diseases without indicating specific types.

[2]Also included a case of herpes.

[3]Included in "colored" section this year.

Source: *MB 1903/04* (1905): 299; *MB 1904/05* (1907): 263; *MB 1905/06* (1907): 324, 327; *MB 1906/07* (1908): 282, 286; *MB 1907/08* (1909): 506, 513; *MB 1908/09* (1910): 472, 475; *MB 1909/10* (1911): 586, 590, 593; *MB 1910/11* (1913): 742; *MB 1911/12* (1915): 616.

Table 18. Frequency of Venereal Diseases in the Navy and Kiautschou Territory, 1897/98 to 1906/07

	Kiautschou	Navy
1897/98	9.26%	11.93%
1898/99	10.25%	12.54%
1899/1900	15.34%	11.00%
1900/01	26.06%	10.54%
1901/02	18.36%	8.18%
1902/03	14.65%	7.64%
1903/04	7.30%	6.68%
1904/05	6.13%	6.24%
1905/06	6.68%	6.49%
1906/07	4.15%	—

Source: Hans Podestà, "Entwicklung und Gestaltung der gesundheitlichen Verhältnisse bei den Besatzungstruppen des Kiautschou-Gebietes . . . ," *Deutsche Militärische Zeitung* 38, no. 4 (1909): 580–581.

Bibliography

Archival Sources

German Federal Archives (BArch)—Berlin-Lichterfelde

Imperial Colonial Office (R1001)

4827 Strafsache gegen Pietro de Grossi (April–July 1908)
4888 Strafsache gegen Josef Scharbatke
4892 Strafsache gegen Dimitris Sametes
5417 Mischehen und Mischlinge—Allgemeines, Bd. 1 (March–November1912)
5671 Lazarettenwesen und Krankenpflege in Ostafrika, Bd. 21 (December1905–April 1924)
5745 Gesundheitsverhältnisse in Deutsch-Ostafrika, Bd. 1 (December 1892–December 1904)
5754 Gesundheitsverhältnisse im deutsch-südwestafrikanischen Schutzgebiete, Bd. 2 (May 1893–February 1900)
5763 Gesundheitsverhältnisse in Kamerun, Bd. 7 (Aug 1909–May 1915)
5764 Gesundheitsverhältnisse in Kamerun, Bd. 8 (June 1913–March 1918)
5765 Gesundheitsverhältnisse in Togo, Bd. 1 (September 1888–November 1902)
5766 Gesundheitsverhältnisse in Togo, Bd. 2 (January 1903–September 1905)
5771 Gesundheitsverhältnisse in Deutsch-Neuguinea, Bd. 3 (May 1908–August 1910)
5772 Gesundheitsverhältnisse in Deutsch-Neuguinea, Bd. 4 (September 1910–May 1913)
5773 Gesundheitsverhältnisse in Deutsch-Neuguinea, Bd. 5 (January 1914–October 1931)
5775 Gesundheitsverhältnisse auf den Karolinen, Bd. 1 (June 1900–December 1902)
5777 Gesundheitsverhältnisse auf den Karolinen, Bd. 3 (July 1905–December 1908)
5779 Gesundheitsverhältnisse auf den Karolinen, Bd. 5 (January 1912–May 1915)
5787 Gesundheitsverhältnisse auf den Marshall-Inseln, Bd. 4 (October 1906–December 1912)
5788 Gesundheitsverhältnisse auf den Marshall-Inseln, Bd. 4 (January 1913–May 1934)
5962 Massnahmen gegen die Syphilis, v.a. auf den Südseeinseln und in Deutsch-Ostafrika sowie allgemein Untersuchungen und Forschungen (February 1900–February 1919)
6010 Medizinal-Jahresberichte über Deutsch-Südwestafrika (June 1905–June 1920)
6012 Medizinal-Jahresberichte über Kamerun—Material für den Jahresbericht (1908–1910)

6040 Bekämpfung der Geschlechtskrankheiten in den deutschen Kolonien (February 1908–February 1918)
6042 Eingeborenen-Lazarette in DSWA (December 1908–May 1912)

Imperial Government Southwest Africa (R151F)

G.iv.D.1 Sittenpolizei: Massregeln gegen geschlechtliche Ausschweifung, Bd. 1
G.iv.D.2 Sittenpolizei: Massregeln gegen geschlechtliche Ausschweifung, Bd. 1
H.ii.h.i. Gesundheitspolizei
H.ii.h.2 Gesundheitspolizei, Bd. 1
H.ii.h.3 Gesundheitspolizei

Nachlass Hintrager (N1037)

File 8 Tätigkeit beim Gouv. in Windhuk, 1904–1913, 1941

Administration of the German Protectorate Togo (R150F)

FA3/86 Imperial Bezirksamt Lome. Gesundheitswesen
FA3/94 Imperial Bezirksamt Lome btr. Ueberwachung der Prostitution
FA3/134 Imperial Government Togo. Gesundheitswesen
FA3/1252 Bezirksamt Atakpame. Gesundheitswesen

German Colonial Society (R8023)

175 Entsendung deutscher Frauen nach DSWA, Bd.6 (November 1900–March 1907)
186 Entsendung deutscher Frauen und Mädchen nach Kiautschou

German Federal Archives—Military Archives (BArch-MA)—Freiburg

Reichsmarineamt (RM3)

6745 Kiautschou—Gouvernementstätigkeitsberichte, Bd. 1 (1898–1899)
6764 Kiautschou—Gouvernementstätigkeitsberichte, Bd. 21 (1911–1912)
6765 Kiautschou—Gouvernementstätigkeitsberichte, Bd. 22 (1912–1913)
6766 Kiautschou—Gouvernementstätigkeitsberichte, Bd. 23 (1913)
6767 Kiautschou—Gouvernementstätigkeitsberichte, Bd. 24 (1913–1914)
7011 Taetigkeitsberichte des Marine-Stabarztes

National Archives of Australia (NAA)

Imperial Government GNG: Correspondence (G2) (1911–1914)

H13 Einfuhr chinesischer Kulis in Nauru
U17 Regierungsärtzliche Stelle Truk
U24 Regierungsarzt Jaluit

Primary Sources

Arbeiten aus dem kaiserlichen Gesundheitsamte, 1897–1904.

Buchner, Max. *Kamerun: Skizzen und Betrachtungen.* Leipzig: Duncker and Humbolt, 1887.

Ehrlich, Paul, ed. *Abhandlungen über Salvarsan (Ehrlich-Hata Präparat 606) gegen Syphilis.* Munich: J. F. Lehmann's Verlag, 1911.

Ehrlich, Paul, and Sahachiro Hata, *Experimentelle Chemotherapie der Spirillosen (Syphilis, Rückfallfieber, Hühnerspirillose, Frambösie).* Berlin: Springer, 1910.

Erdland, August. *Die Marshall-Insulaner. Leben und Sitte, Sinn und Religion eines Südsee-Volkes.* Munster: Aschendorffsche Verlagsbuchhandlung, 1914.

Erzberger, Matthias. *Die Kolonial-Bilanz. Bilder aus der deutschen Kolonialpolitik auf Grund der Verhandlungen des Reichstags im Sessionsabschnitt 1905/06.* Berlin: Germania, 1906.

Heim, Gustav. "Die Syphilis in den deutschen Schutzgebieten." *Archiv für Dermatologie und Syphilis* 118 (1913): 165–198.

Hintze, K. "Welchen Einfluß hat das Tropenklima auf Angehörige der weißen Rasse?" *ASTH* 20, no. 6 (1916): 91–104.

Hoffmann, Albert. *Lebenserinnerungen eines Rheinischen Missionars,* vol 1: *Auf dem Missionsfeld in Neu-Guinea.* Wuppertal: Verlag der Rheinischen Missionsgesellschaft, 1948.

Jäger. "Beiträge zur Rassenhygiene aus dem Bezirk Ebolowa (Südkamerun)." *ASTH* 16, no. 10 (1910): 325–336.

Kersten, Hans. "Die Gonorrhöe im Bezirk Rabaul (Deutsch-Neuguinea)," *Beihefte zum ASTH* 29 (1925): 180–189.

Kohlbrugge J. H. F. 1900, "Syphilis in den Kolonien." *ASTH* 4, no. 4 (1900): 219.

Kohlstock, Paul. *Ratgeber für die Tropen. Handbuch für Ausrüstung, Aufenthalt, Reisen und Behandlung von Krankheiten,* 3rd ed. Stettin: Hermann Peters Verlag, 1910.

———. "Ueber die Dienstverhältnisse der in den deutschen Schutzgebieten beamteten Aerzte. "*Deutsche medizinische Wochenschrift* 25 (1899): 33–35.

Kronecker, Franz. "Fünfzehn Jahre Kiautschou," *Deutsche Medizinische Presse* (1913): 1–31.

Külz, Ludwig. *Blätter und Briefe eines eines Arztes aus dem tropischen Deutschafrika.* Berlin: Wilhelm Süsserott, 1906.

———. "Grundzüge der kolonialen Eingeborenenhygiene," *Beihefte zum ASTH* 15 (1911): 1–95.

Leutwein, Theodor. *Elf Jahre Gouverneur in Deutsch-Südwestafrika.* Berlin: Mittler and Sohn, 1906.

Medizinal-Berichte über die Deutschen Schutzgebiete, 1905–1906 to 1913.

Mense, C. 1900, "Syphilis und venerische Krankheiten in den neu der Kultur erschlossenen Ländern besonders Afrika." *ASTH* 4, no. 2 (1900): 86–109.

Podestà, Hans. "Entwicklung und Gestaltung der gesundheitlichen Verhältnisse bei den Besatzungstruppen des Kiautschou-Gebietes im Vergleich mit der Marine und unter besonderer Berücksichtigung von Örtlichkeit und Klima in Tsingtau." *Deutsche Militärische Zeitschrift* 38, no. 14 (1909): 569–601.

Reichskolonialamt, ed. *Die deutschen Schutzgebiete in Afrika und der Südsee 1912/1913. Amtliche Jahresberichte.* Berlin: Mittler, 1914.

Reiner, Otto. *Achtzehn Jahre Farmer in Afrika.* Leipzig: Paul List Verlag, 1924.

Schilling, Claus. "Über den ärztlchen Dienst in den deutschen Schutzgebieten." *Beihefte zum ASTH* 13, no. 6 (1909): 33–45.

Scheube, B. "Die venerische Krankheiten in den warmen Ländern." *ASTH* 6, no. 5 (1902): 147–160.

———. "Die venerische Krankheiten in den warmen Ländern (Fortsetzung)." *ASTH* 6, no. 6 (1902): 187–207.

———. "Die venerische Krankheiten in den warmen Ländern (Fortsetzung und Schluss)." *ASTH* 6, no. 7 (1902): 219–244.

Seiner, Franz. *Bergtouren und Steppenfahrten im Hererolande.* Berlin: Wilhem Süsserott, 1904.
Steudel, Emil. "Der ärztliche Dienst in den deutschen Schutzgebieten." *Beihefte zum ASTH* 13, no. 6 (1909): 17–31.
Uthemann and Fürth. "Tsingtau: Ein kolonialhygienischer Einblick auf die Entwicklung des Deutschen Kiautschougebiets." *Beihefte zum ASTH* 15 (1911): 5–39.
Vargyas, Gàbor. *Data on the Pictorial History of North-East Papua New Guinea.* Budapest: Ethnographical Institute of the Hungarian Academy of Sciences, 1986.
Verhandlungen des Reichtags, 1912, vol. 238. http://www.reichstagsprotokolle.de/Blatt_k13_bsb00003350_00106.html.
Vieweg, Burkhard. *Big Fellow Man. Muschelgeld und Südseegeister. Authentische Berichte aus Deutsch-Neuguinea 1906–1909.* Weikersheim: Margraf, 1990.
———. *Macho Porini. Die Augen im Busch. Kauschukpflanzer Karl Vieweg in Deutsch-Ostafrika Authentische Berichte 1910–1919.* Weikersheim: Markgraf Verlag, 1996.
von Spiegel, E. Freiherr. *Meere, Inseln, Menschen. Vom Seekadetten zum U-Boot-Kommandanten.* Berlin: August Scherl, 1934.
Werner, H. "Die Organisation des Sanitätsdienstes in den ehemaligen deutschen Schutzgebieten vor und nach dem Weltkriege." *Deutsche medizinische Wochenschrift* 64 (1938): 268–271, 309–313.
Wechselmann, Wilhelm. *The Treatment of Syphilis with Salvarsan.* Translated by Abraham Wolbarst, New York: Rebman, 1911.
Zechmeister, Hugo. "Die Syphilis in den Tropen, deren Verlauf und Behandlung." *ASTH* 12, no. 11 (1908): 350–359.
Ziemann, Hans. "Über die Errichtung von Tropeninstituten und die Gestaltung des ärzlichen Dienstes in den deutschen Schutzgebieten." *Beihefte zum ASTH* 13, no. 6 (1909): 46–54.
———. *Wie erobert man Afrika für die weiße und farbige Rasse?* Leipzig: Barth, 1907.

Secondary Sources

Abrams, Lynn. "Prostitutes in Imperial Germany, 1870–1918: Working Girls or Social Outcasts?" In *The German Underworld: Deviants and Outcasts in German History,* ed. Richard Evans, 189–209. London: Routledge, 1988.
Adas, Michael. "From Avoidance to Confrontation: Peasant Protest in Precolonial and Colonial Southeast Asia." *Comparative Studies in Society and History* 23, no. 2 (1981): 217–247.
Akyeampong, Emmanuel. *Drink, Power, and Cultural Change: A Social History of Alcohol in Ghana c. 1900 to Recent Times.* Portsmouth, NH: Heinemann, 1996.
Arnold, David. *Colonizing the Body: State Medicine and Epidemic Disease in Nineteenth-Century India.* Berkeley: University of California Press, 1993.
———. '"Public Health and Public Power: Medicine and Hegemony in Colonial India." In *Contesting Colonial Hegemony: State and Society in Africa and India,* ed. Dagmar Engels and Shula Marks, 131–151. London: British Academic Press, 1994.
Asad, Talal. "Ethnographic Representation, Statistics, and Modern Power." In *From the Margins: Historical Anthropology and Its Futures,* ed. Brian Axel, 66–91. Durham, NC: Duke University Press, 2002.

Asiwaju, A. I. "Migration as Revolt: The examples of Ivory Coast and Upper Volta before 1945." *Journal of African History* 14 (1976): 577–594.

Becher, Jürgen. *Dar es Salaam, Tanga und Tabora. Stadtentwicklung in Tansania unter deutscher Kolonialherrschaft (1885–1914).* Stuttgart: Franz Steiner, 1997.

Biener, Annette. *Das deutsche Pachgebiet Tsingtau in Schantung, 1897–1914: Institutioneller Wandel durch Kolonialisierung.* Bonn: Matzat, 2001.

Blackbourn, David. "The German Bourgeoisie: An Introduction." In *The German Bourgeoisie: Essays on the Social History of the German Middle Class from the Late Eighteenth to the Early Twentieth Century,* ed. David Blackbourn and Richard Evans, 1–45. London: Routledge, 1991.

Bleys, Rudi. *The Geography of Perversion: Mate-to-male Sexual Behaviour outside the West and the Ethnographic Imagination, 1750–1918.* New York: New York University Press, 1995.

Bonner, Phil. "'Desirable or undesirable Basotho women?' Liquor, prostitution and migration of Basotho women to the Rand, 1920–1945." In *Women and Gender in Southern Africa to 1945,* ed. Cheryl Walker, 221–250. Claremont, South Africa: David Philip Publishers, 1990.

Bozzoli, Belinda. *Women of Phokeng: Consciousness, Life Strategy, and Migrancy in South Africa, 1900–1933.* Portsmouth, NH: Heinemann, 1991.

Breuilly, John. "Urbanization and social transformation, 1800–1914." In *Germany: A New Social and Economic History,* vol. 3, *Since 1800,* ed. Scheilagh Ogilvie and Richard Overy, 192–226. London: Arnold, 2003.

Bühler, Andreas. *Der Namaaufstand gegen die deutsche Kolonialherrschaft in Namibia von 1904 bis 1913.* Frankfurt: IKO, Verlag für Interkulturelle Kommunikation, 2003.

Bullough, Vern, and Bonnie Bullough. *Women and Prostitution: A Social History.* Buffalo, NY: Prometheus Books, 1987 (1978).

Burleigh, Michael, and Wolfgang Wippermann. *The Racial State: Germany 1933–1945.* New York: Cambridge University Press, 1991.

Castles, Stephen. "Migrant Settlement, Transnational Communities and State Strategies in the Asia Pacific Region." In *Migration in the Asia Pacific: Population, Settlement and Citizenship Issues,* ed. Robyn Iredale, Charles Hawksley, and Stephen Castles, 3–26. Northampton, MA: Edward Elgar, 2003.

Conklin, Alice. "Redefining 'Frenchness': Citizenship, Race Regeneration, and Imperial Motherhood in France and West Africa, 1914–40." In *Domesticating the Empire: Race, Gender, and Family Life in French and Dutch Colonialism,* ed. Julia Clancy-Smith and Frances Gouda, 65–83. Charlottesville: University of Virginia Press, 1988.

Connell, R. W. *Gender and Power: Society, the Person and Sexual Politics.* Stanford, CA: Stanford University Press, 1987.

———. *Masculinities.* Berkeley: University of California Press, 1995.

Conrad, Sebastion. *Globalisation and the Nation in Imperial Germany.* Cambridge: Cambridge University Press, 2010.

Conrad, Sebastian, and Shalini Randeria, "Geteilte Geschichten: Europa in einer postkolonialen Welt." In *Jenseits des Eurozentrismus: Postkoloniale Perspektiven in den Geschichts- und Kulturwissenschaften,* ed. Conrad and Randeria, 9–49. Frankfurt: Campus, 2002.

Davidson, Raelene. "'As good a bloody woman as any other woman …': Prostitutes in Western Australia, 1895–1939." In *Exploring Women's Pasts: Essays in Social History,* ed. Patricia Crawford and Margaret Anderson, 171–201. London: Allen & Unwin, 1984.

Davies, Margit. "Das Gesundheitswesen im Kaiser-Wilhelmsland und im Bismarckarchipel." In *Die deutsche Südsee 1884–1914. Ein Handbuch,* ed. Hermann Hiery, 417–449. Paderborn: Ferdinand Schönigh, 2001.

———. *Public Health and Colonialism: The Case of German New Guinea 1884–1914.* Wiesbaden: Harrassowitz Verlag, 2002.

Debusmann, Robert. "Krankheit im kolonialen Alltag: Ärtzliche Erfahrungen und Patientenverhalten in Kamerun, 1890–1930." In *Afrika und die Globalisierung,* ed. Hans Peter Hahn and Gerd Spittler, 217–225. Münster: Lit, 1999.

De Groot, Joanna. "'Sex' and 'Race': The Construction of Language and Image in the Nineteenth Century." In *Sexuality and Subordination: Interdisciplinary Studies of Gender in the Nineteenth Century,* ed. Susan Mendus and Jane Rendall, 89–128. London: Routledge, 1989.

Delancey, Mark. "Health and Disease on the Plantations of Cameroon, 1884–1939." In *Disease in Africa: An Introductory Survey and Case Studies,* ed. David Patterson and Gerald Hartwig, 153–179. Durham, NC: Duke University Press, 1978.

Drechsler Hans. *Let Us Die Fighting: the Struggle of the Herero and the Name against German imperialism (1884–1915),* 3rd ed. Berlin: Akademie Verlag, 1986.

Dreyfus, Hubert, and Paul Rabinow, *Michel Foucault: Beyond Structuralism and Hermeneutics.* Brighton: Harvester Press, 1982.

Eckart, Wolfgang. "Arzneimittelerprobung in der ehemaligen deutschen Kolonie Togo." *Forum Wissenschaft* 1 (1988): 29–35.

———. *Medizin und Kolonialimperialismus: Deutschland 1884–1945.* Paderborn: Ferdinand Schönigh, 1997.

———. "Medicine and German colonial expansion in the Pacific: the Caroline, Mariana, and Marshall Islands." In *Disease, Medicine, and Empire: Perspectives on Western Medicine and the Experience of European Expansion,* ed. Roy Macleod and Milton Lewis, 80–102. London: Routledge, 1988.

Eckert, Andreas. *Die Duala und die Kolonialmächte: Eine Untersuchung zu Widerstand, Protest und Protonationalismus in Kamerun vor dem Zweiten Weltkrieg.* Münster: Lit, 1991.

———. *Grundbesitz, Landkonflikte und kolonialer Wandel: Douala 1880 bis 1960.* Stuttgart: Franz Steiner, 1999.

Elkeles, Barbara. *Der moralische Diskurs über das medizinische Menschenexperimente im 19. Jahrhundert.* Stuttgart: Gustav Fischer, 1996.

El-Tayeb, Fatima. *Schwarze Deutsche: Der Diskurs um "Rasse" und nationale Identität 1890–1933.* Frankfurt: Campus, 2001.

———. "Verbotene Begegnungen—unmögliche Existenzen. Afrikanisch-deutsche Beziehungen und Afro-Deutsche im Spannungsfeld von *race* and *gender.*" In *Die (koloniale) Begegnung. AfrikanerInnen in Deutschland 1880–1945. Deutsche in Afrika 1880–1918,* ed. Marianne Bechhaus-Gerst and Reinhard Klein-Arendt, 85–95. Frankfurt: Peter Lang, 2003.

Essner, Claudia. "'Wo Rauch ist, da ist auch Feuer:' Zu den Ansätzen eines Rassenrechts für die Deutschen Kolonien." In *Rassendiskriminierung, Kolonialpolitik und ethnisch-nationale Identität. Referate des 2. Internationalen Kolonialgeschichtlichen Symposiums 1991 in Berlin,* ed. Wilfried Wagner, 145–160. Hamburg: Lit, 1992.

Evans, Richard. "Family and class in the Hamburg grand bourgeoisie, 1815–1914." In *The German Bourgeoisie: Essays on the Social History of the German Middle Class from the late eighteenth to the early twentieth Century,* ed. David Blackbourn and Richard Evans, 115–139. London: Routledge, 1991.

———. "Introduction: The 'Dangerous Classes' in Germany from the Middle Ages to the Twentieth Century." In *The German Underworld: Deviants and Outcasts in German History*, ed. Richard Evans, 1–28. London: Routledge, 1988.
———. "Prostitution, State and Society in Imperial Germany." *Past and Present* 70 (1976): 106–129.
Eves, Richard. "Unsettling settler colonialism: Debates over climate and colonization in New Guinea, 1875–1914." *Ethnic and Racial Studies* 28, no. 2 (2005): 304–330.
Fanon, Franz. *Black Skin, White Masks.* New York: Grove Press, 1982.
"Feminist Perspectives on Objectification." *Stanford Encyclopedia of Philosophy.* 10 March 2010, revised 28 June 2011. http://www.plato.stanford.edu/entries/feminism-objectification/ (accessed 19 September 2011).
Firth, Stewart. *New Guinea under the Germans.* Carlton: Melbourne University Press, 1983.
Fleck, Ludwik. *Genesis and Development of a Scientific Fact.* Chicago: University of Chicago Press, 1979.
Foucault, Michel. *The Archaeology of Knowledge.* New York: Pantheon Books, 1972.
———. *The Birth of Biopolitics: Lectures at the Collège de France. 1978–1979,* ed. Michel Senellart. Houndsmill, NH: Palgrave Macmillan, 2008.
———. *Discipline and Punish: The Birth of the Prison.* New York: Pantheon Books, 1977.
———. *The History of Sexuality: An Introduction.* New York: Vintage Books, 1990.
Frances, Raelene. "Sex Workers or Citizens? Prostitution and the Shaping of 'Settler' Society in Australia." *International Review of Social History* 44 (1999): 101–122.
Frevert, Ute. "Professional Medicine and the Working Classes in Imperial Germany." *Journal of Contemporary History* 20 (1985): 637–658.
Gilman, Sander. "Black Sexuality and Modern Consciousness." In *Blacks and German Culture,* ed. Reinhold Grimm and Jost Hermand, 35–53. Madison: University of Wisconsin Press, 1986.
———. "Black Bodies, White Bodies: Toward an Iconography of Female Sexuality in Late Nineteenth-Century Art, Medicine, and Literature." *Critical Inquiry* 12, no. 1 (1985): 204–242.
———. *Difference and Pathology: Stereotypes of Sexuality, Race, and Madness.* Ithaca, NY: Cornell University Press, 1985.
Göckenjan, Gerd. *Kurien und Staat machen: Gesundheit und Medizin in der bürgerlichen Welt.* Frankfurt: Suhrkamp, 1985.
———. "Wandlungen im Selbstbild des Arztes seit dem 19. Jahrhundert." In *Medizinische Deutungsmacht im sozialen Wandel des 19. und frühen 20. Jahrhunderts,* edited by Alfons Labish and Reinhard Spree, 89–102. Bonn: Psychatrie-Verlag, 1989.
Goos, Philipp. "Bubo." Jameda. 2007–2012; last update 2 March 2012. http://www.jameda.de/medikamente/krankheiten/tropischer-bubo/a55_4209/ (accessed 11 April 2012).
Grosse, Pascal. *Kolonialismus, Eugenik und bürgerliche Gesellschaft in Deutschland 1850–1918.* Frankfurt: Campus, 2000.
———. "Turning Native? Anthropology, German Colonialism, and the Paradoxes of the 'Acclimatization Question,' 1885–1914." In *Worldly Provincialism: German Anthropology in the Age of Empire,* ed. H. Glenn Penny and Matti Bunzl, 192–196. Ann Arbor: The University of Michigan Press, 2003.
Gründer, Horst. *Christliche Mission und deutscher Imperialismus. Eine politische Geschichte ihrer Beziehungen während der deutschen Kolonialzeit (1884–1914) unter besonderer Berücksichtigung Afrikas und Chinas.* Paderborn: Ferdinand Schöningh, 1982.

———. *Geschichte der deutschen Kolonien.* Paderborn: Ferdinand Schönigh, 1991.

Grüntzig, Johannes, and Heinz Mehlhorn. *Expeditionen ins Reich der Seuchen: Medizinische Himmelfahrtskommando der deutschen Kaiser- und Kolonialzeit.* Munich: Spektrum, 2005.

Hartmann, Wolfram. "Sexual Encounters and Their Implications on an Open and Closing Frontier: Central Namibia from the 1840s to 1905." PhD dissertation, Columbia University, 2002.

———. "Eine *situation érotique et coloniale* im 19. Jahrhundert: Männer und Frauen im südwestlichen Afrika." In *Die (koloniale) Begegnung. AfrikanerInnen in Deutschland 1880–1945. Deutsche in Afrika 1880–1918,* ed. Marianne Bechhaus-Gerst and Reinhard Klein-Arendt, 129–145. Frankfurt: Peter Lang, 2003.

———. "Urges in the colony: Men and women in colonial Windhoek, 1890–1914." *Journal of Namibian Studies* 1 (2007): 39–71.

Hausen, Karin. "Family and Role-Division: The Polarisation of Sexual Stereotypes in the Nineteenth Century—An Aspect of the Dissociation of Work and Family Life." In *The German Family: Essays on the Social History of the Family in Nineteenth- and Twentieth-Century Germany,* ed. Richard Evans and W. R. Lees, 51–83. London: Groom Helm, 1981.

Hawkins, Sean. *Writing and Colonialism in Northern Ghana: The Encounter between the LoDagga and "the World on Paper."* Toronto: Toronto University Press, 2002.

Hempenstall, Peter. *Pacific Islanders under German Rule: A Study in the Meaning of Colonial Resistance.* Canberra: Australian National University Press, 1978.

Hempenstall, Peter, and Noel Rutherford. *Protest and Dissent in the Colonial Pacific.* Suva: Institute of Pacific Studies of the University of the South Pacific, 1984.

Henderson, W. O. *Studies in German Colonial History.* Chicago: Quadrangle Books, 1962.

Henriot, Christian. *Prostitution and Sexuality in Shanghai: A Social History, 1849–1949.* Trans. Noël Castelino. Cambridge: Cambridge University Press, 2001.

Hershatter, Gail. *Dangerous Pleasures: Prostitution and Modernity in Twentieth-Century Shanghai.* Berkeley: University of California Press, 1997.

Hesselink, Liesbeth. "Prostitution: A 'Necessary Evil,' Particularly in the Colonies. Views on Prostitution in the Netherlands Indies." In *Indonesian Women in Focus: Past and Present Notions,* ed. Elsbeth Locher-Scholten and Anke Niehof, 205–224. Dardrecht, Holland: Foris Publications, 1987.

Hiery, Hermann. *Das Deutsche Reich in der Südsee (1900–1921). Eine Annäherung an die Erfahrungen verschiedener Kulturen.* Göttingen: Vandenhoeck & Ruprecht, 1995.

———, ed. *Die deutsche Südsee: 1884–1914: Ein Handbuch.* Paderborn: Schönigh, 2001.

———. "Germans, Pacific Islanders and Sexuality: German Impact and Indigenous Influence in Melanesia and Micronesia." In *European Impact and Pacific Influence: British and German Colonial Policy in the Pacific Islands and the Indigenous Response,* ed. Herman Hiery and John MacKenzie, 299–323. London: Tauris Academic Studies, 1997.

Hilpert-Fröhlich, Christiana. *"Auf zum Kampfe wider die Unzucht." Prostitution und Sittlichkeitsbewegung in Essen 1890–1914.* Bochum: SWI-Verlag, 1991.

Howell, Philip. *Geographies of Regulation: Policing Prostitution in nineteenth-century Britain and the Empire.* Cambridge: Cambridge University Press, 2009.

Huang, Fu-the. *Qingdao: Chinesen unter deutscher Herrschaft 1897–1914.* Bochum: Projekt, 1999.

Hull, Isabel. *Sexuality, State, and Civil Society in Germany, 1700–1815.* Ithaca, NY: Cornell University Press, 1996.

Hulverscheidt, Marion. "German Malariology Experiments with Humans: Supported by the DFG until 1945." In *Man, Medicine, and the State: The Human Body as an Object of Government Sponsored Medical Research in the 20th Century,* ed. Wolfgang Eckart, 225–229. Stuttgart: Franz Steiner Verlag, 2006.

Hüntelmann, Axel. "1910. Transformationen eines Arzneistoffes—vom 606 zum Salvarsan." In *Arzneimittel des 20. Jahrhunderts: 13 historische Skizzen von Lebertran bis Contergan,* ed. Nicholas Eschenbruch et al., 17–51. Bielefeld: Transcript, 2009.

———. *Hygiene im Namen des Staates: Das Reichsgesundheitsamt 1876–1933.* Göttingen: Wallstein, 2008.

———. "Zwischen Kooperation und Kontrolle." In *Gesundheit und Staat: Studien zur Geschichte der Gesundheitsämter in Deutschland, 1870–1950,* ed. Axel Hüntelmann, Johannes Vossen, and Herwig Czech, 27–48. Husum: Matthiesen, 2006.

Huerkamp, Claudia. "Ärzte und Patienten: Zum strukturellen Wandel der Arzt-Patient-Beziehung vom ausgehenden 18. Bis zum frühen 20. Jahrhundert." In *Medizinische Deutungsmacht im sozialen Wandel des 19. und frühen 20. Jahrhunderts,* ed. Alfons Labish and Reinhard Spree, 57–73. Bonn: Psychatrie-Verlag, 1989.

———. *Der Austieg der Ärzte im 19. Jahrhundert. Vom gelehrten Stand zum professionellen Experten: Das Beispiel Preußens.* Göttingen: Vandenhoeck and Ruprecht, 1985.

———. "The Making of the Modern Medical Profession, 1800–1914: Prussian Doctors in the Nineteenth Century." In *German Professions, 1800–1950,* ed. Geoffrey Cooks and Konrad Jarausch, 66–84. New York: Oxford University Press, 1990.

———. "Die preussisch-deutsche Ärzteschaft als Teil des Bildungsbürgertums." In *Bildungsbürgertum im 19. Jahrhundert,* vol. I, *Bildungssystem und Professionalisierung in internationalen Vergleich,* ed. Werner Conze and Jürgen Kocka, 358–387. Stuttgart: Klett-Cotta, 1985.

Hyam, Ronald. *Empire and Sexuality: The British Experience.* Manchester: Manchester University Press, 1990.

Iliffe, John. *Tanganyika under German Rule, 1905–1912.* London: Cambridge University Press, 1969.

Isobe, Hiroyuki. *Medizin und Kolonialismus: Die Bekämpfung der Schlafkrankheit in den deutschen "Schutzgebieten" vor dem Ersten Weltkrieg.* Berlin: Lit Verlag, 2009.

Jenders, Andrea, and Andreas Müller, *"Nur die Dummen sind eingeschrieben …": Dortmunder Dirnen- und Sittengeschichte zwischen 1870 und 1927.* Dortumund: Geschichtswerkstatt Dortmund: 1993.

Jochelson, Karen. "Sexually Transmitted Diseases in Nineteenth- and Twentieth-Century South Africa." In *Histories of Sexually Transmitted Diseases and HIV/AIDS in Sub-Saharan Africa,* ed. Philip Setel, Milton Lewis, and Maryinez Lyons, 219–243. Westport, CT: Greenwood Press, 1999.

———. "Tracking Down the Treponema: Patterns of Syphilis in South Africa, 1880—1940." STRUCTURE AND EXPERIENCE IN THE MAKING OF APARTHEID, History Workshop, University of Witwatersrand. Accessed through WIReDSpace, University of Witwatersrand, Johannesburg, 2002–2011. http://wiredspace.wits.ac.za/bitstream/handle/10539/7881/HWS-202.pdf?sequence=1 (accessed 12 April 2012).

Kapoor, Ilan. *The Postcolonial Politics of Development.* Oxon: Routledge, 2008.

Kenosian, David. "The Colonial Body Politic: Desire and Violence in the Works of Gustav Frenssen and Hans Grimm." *Monatshefte* 89 (1997): 182–195.

Kertzer, David, and Dominique Arel. "Censuses, Identity Formation, and the Struggle for Political Power." In *Census and Identity: The Politics of Race, Ethnicity, and Language in National Censuses,* ed. David Kertzer and Dominique Arel, 1–42. Cambridge: Cambridge University Press, 2002.

Kevles, Daniel. *In the Name of Eugenics: Genetics and the Uses of Human Heredity.* New York: Alfred Knopf, 1985.

Klein, Thoralf. "Rasse—Kultur—soziale Stellung: Konzeptionen des 'Eingeborenen' und koloniale Segregation in Kiautschou." In *Rassenmischehen—Mischlinge—Rassentrennung. Zur Politik der Rasse im deutsch Kolonialreich,* ed. Franz Becker, 304–328. Stuttgart: Steiner Verlag, 2004.

Knoll, Arthur. "Decision-Making for the German Colonies." In *Germans in the Tropics: Essays in German Colonial History,* ed. Arthur Knoll and Lewis Gann, 131–149. New York: Greenwood Press, 1987.

———. *Togo under Imperial Germany 1884–1914.* Stanford, CA: Hoover Institution Press, 1978.

Koponen, Juhani. *Development for Exploitation: German Colonial Policies in Mainland Tanzania, 1884–1914.* Helsinki: Tiedekirja, 1995.

Krüger, Gesine. *Kriegsbewältigung und Geschichtsbewußtsein. Realität, Deutung und Verarbeitung des deutschen Kolonialkrieges in Namibia 1904 bis 1907.* Göttingen: Vandenhoeck and Ruprecht, 1999.

Kundrus, Birthe. *Moderne Imperialisten. Das Kaiserreich im Spiegel seiner Kolonien.* Cologne: Böhlau, 2003.

———. "'Weiß und herrlich': Überlegungen zu einer Geschlechtergeschichte des Kolonialismus." In *Projektionen. Rassismus und Sexismus in der Visuellen Kultur,* ed. Annegrete Friedrich et al., 41–50. Marburg: Jonas Verlag, 1997.

Labisch, Alfons. "Doctors, Workers and the Scientific Cosmology of the Industrial World: The Social Construction of 'Health' and the 'Homo Hygienicus.'" *Journal of Contemporary History* 20 (1985): 599–615

———. "From Traditional Individualism to Collective Professionalism: State, Patient, Compulsory Health Insurance, and the Panel Doctor Question in Germany, 1883–1931." In *Medicine and Modernity: Public Health and Medical Care in Nineteenth- and Twentieth-Century Germany,* ed. Manfred Berg and Geoffrey Cooks, 35–54. Washington, DC: German Historical Institute, 1997.

———. "Gesundheitskonzepte und Medizin im Prozeß der Zivilisation." In *Medizinisch Deutungsmacht Medizinische Deutungsmacht im sozialen Wandel des 19. und frühen 20. Jahrhunderts,* ed. Alfons Labish and Reinhard Spree, 15–36. Bonn: Psychatrie-Verlag, 1989.

Lachmund, Jens, and Gunnar Stollberg. *Patientenwelten: Krankheit und Medizin vom späten 18. bis zum frühen 20. Jahrhundert im Spiegel von Autobiographien.* Opladen: Leske und Budrich, 1995.

Leven, Karl-Heinz. *Die Geschichte der Infektionskrankheiten: Von der Antike bis ins 20. Jahrhundert.* Landsberg and Lech: ecomed, 1997.

Levine, Philippa. "'A Multitude of Unchaste Women:' Prostitution in the British Empire." *Journal of Women's History* 14, no. 4 (2004): 159–163.

———. *Prostitution, Race and Politics: Policing Venereal Disease in the British Empire.* New York: Routledge, 2003.

Lewis, Milton, and Scott Bamber. "Introduction." In *Sex, Disease, and Society: A Comparative History of Sexually Transmitted Diseases and HIV/AIDS in Asia and the Pacific,* ed. Milton Lewis, Scott Bamber, and Michael Waugh, 1–17. Westport, CT: Greenwood Press, 1997.

Little, Kenneth. *African Women in Towns: An Aspect of Africa's Social Revolution.* Cambridge: Cambridge University Press, 1973.

Mair, Lucy. *African Marriage and Social Change.* London: Frank Cass & Co, 1969.

Malinowski, B. "Kula: The Circulating Exchange of Valuable in the Archipelagoes of Eastern New Guinea." In *Peoples of the Pacific: The History of Oceania to 1870,* ed. Paul D'Arcy, 261–270. Burlington, VT: Ashgate/Variorum, 2008.

Mamozai, Martha. *Schwarze Frau, weiße Herrin. Frauenleben in den deutschen Kolonien.* Reinbek: Rowohlt, 1989.

McClelland, Charles. *The German Experience of Professionalization: Modern learned professions and their organizations from the early nineteenth to the Hitler era.* Cambridge: Cambridge University Press, 1991.

———. "Modern German Doctors: A Failure of Professionalization." In *Medicine and Modernity: Public Health and Medical Care in Nineteenth- and Twentieth-Century Germany,* ed. Manfred Berg and Geoffrey Cocks, 81–97. Washington, DC: German Historical Institute, 1997.

McCulloch, Jock. "The Management of Venereal Disease in Settler Society: Colonial Zimbabwe, 1900–30," In *Histories of Sexually Transmitted Diseases and HIV/AIDS in Sub-Saharan Africa,* ed. Philip Setel, Milton Lewis, and Maryinez Lyons, 195–216. Westport, CT: Greenwood Press, 1999.

Michels, Stefanie. "Soldatische Frauenwelten." In *Frauen in den deutschen Kolonien,* ed. Marianne Bechhaus-Gerst and Mechthild Leutner, 122–130. Berlin: Ch. Links, 2009.

Ming, Hannecke. "Barracks-Concubinage in the Indies, 1887–1920." *Indonesia* 35 (1983): 63–93.

Mosse, George. *Nationalism and Sexuality: Respectability and Abnormal Sexuality in Modern Europe.* New York: Howard Fertig, 1985.

———. *Toward the Final Solution: A History of European Racism.* New York: Howard Fertig, 1985 (1978).

Mühlhahn, Klaus. *Herrschaft und Widerstand in der "Musterkolonie" Kiautschou: Interaktionen zwischen China und Deutschland, 1897–1914.* Munich: Oldenburg, 2000.

Musambachime, M. C. "Protest Migrations in Mweru-Luapula 1900–1940." *African Studies* 47 (1988): 19–34.

Neill, Deborah. "Transnationalism in the Colonies: Cooperation, Rivalry, and Race in German and French Tropical Medicine." PhD dissertation, University of Toronto, 2005.

Noyes, John. *Colonial Space. Spatiality in the discourse of German South West Africa 1884–1915.* Chur: Harwood Academic Publishers, 1992.

———. "Wide Open Spaces and the Hunger for Land: Production of Space in the German Colonial Novel." *Faultline: Interdisciplinary Approaches to German Studies* 1 (1992): 103–117.

Nuhn, Walter. *Kamerun unter dem Kaiseradler: Geschichte der Erwerbung und Erschliessung des ehemaligen deutschen Schutzgebietes Kamerun: ein Beitrag zur deutschen Kolonialgeschichte.* Dessau: Wilhelm Herbst, 2000.

O'Donnell, Krista. "The Colonial Woman Question: Gender, National Identity, and Empire in the German Colonial Society Female Emigration Program, 1896–1914." PhD dissertation, SUNY Binghamton, 1996.

Oermann, Nils. *Mission, Church and State Relations in South West Africa under German Rule (1884–1914).* Stuttgart: Franz Steiner Verlag, 1999.

Oloukpona-Yinnon, Adjaï Paulin. "Zur Begegnung zwischen Weiß und Schwarz in Deutschland im kolonialen Kontext. Das Beispiel von Togoern im kaiserlichen Deutschland." In *Die (koloniale) Begegnung. AfrikanerInnen in Deutschland 1880–1945. Deutsche in Afrika 1880–1918,* ed. Marianne Bechhaus-Gerst and Reinhard Klein-Arendt, 237–254. Frankfurt: Peter Lang, 2003.

Oriel, J. D. *The Scars of Venus: A History of Venereology.* London: Springer-Verlag, 1994.

Pabst, Martin. *Mission und Kolonialpolitik: Die Norddeutsche Missionsgesellschaft an der Goldküste und in Togo bis zum Ausbruck des Ersten Weltkrieges.* Munich: Anarche, 1988.

Pandey, Gyanendra. "Voices from the Edge: The Struggle to Write Subaltern Histories." In *Mapping Subaltern Studies and the Postcolonial,* ed. Vinayak Chaturvedi, 281–299. London: Verso, 2000.

Peers, Douglas. "Contours of the Garrison State: The Army and the Historiography of Early Nineteenth-Century India." In *Orientalism, Evangelicalism and the Military Cantonment in Early Nineteenth-Century India: A Historiographical Overview,* ed. Nancy Cassels, 89–123. Lewiston: Edwin Mellon Press, 1991.

Peukert, Detlev. *Inside Nazi Germany: Conformity, Opposition, and Racism in Everyday Life.* New Haven, CT: Yale University Press, 1987.

Pierard, Richard. "The Transportation of White Women to German Southwest Africa, 1898–1914." *Race* (1970–1971): 317–322.

Prein, Philipp. "Guns and Top Hats: African Resistance in German South West Africa, 1907–1915." *Journal of Southern African Studies* 20, no. 1 (1994): 99–121.

Prins, Gwyn. "Review Article: But what was the disease? The present state of health and healing in African Studies." *Past and Present* 124 (1989): 159–179.

Proctor, Robert. *Racial Hygiene: Medicine under the Nazis.* Cambridge, MA: Harvard University Press, 1988.

Randeria, Shalini. "Geteilte Geschichte und verwobene Moderne." In *Zukunftsentwürfe: Ideen für eine Kultur der Veränderung,* ed. Jörn Rüsen, Hanna Leitgab, and Norbert Jegelka, 87–96. Frankfurt: Campus, 2000.

Regin, Cornelia. "Zwischen Angriff und Abwehr: Die Naturheilbewegung als medizinkritische Öffentlichkeit im Deutschen Kaiserreich." In *Medizinkritische Bewegungen im Deutschen Reich (ca. 1870–ca. 1933),* ed. Marin Dinges, 39–58. Stuttgart: Franz Steiner Verlag, 1996.

Rudin, Harry. *Germans in the Cameroons 1884–1914: A Case Study in Modern Imperialism.* New Haven, CT: Yale University Press, 1938.

Sabisch, Katja. *Das Weib als Versuchsperson: Medizinische Menschenexperimente im 19. Jahrhundert am Beispiel der Syphilisforschung.* Bielefeld: Transcript, 2007.

Sack, Peter, and Dymphna Clark, ed. and trans. *German New Guinea: The Annual Reports.* Canberra: Australian National University Press, 1979.

Sadj, Amadou Booker. *Das Bild des Negro-Afrikaners in der Deutschen Kolonialliteratur (1884–1945). Ein Beitrag zur literarischen Imagologie Schwarzafrikas.* Berlin: Dietrich Reimer Verlag, 1985.

Said, Edward. *Orientalism.* New York: Vintage Books, 1979.

Samulski, Roland. "Die 'Sünde' im Auge des Betrachters—Rassenmischung und deutsche Rassenpolitik im Schutzgebiet Samoa 1900 bis 1914." In *Rassenmischehen—Misch-*

linge—Rassentrennung. Zur Politik der Rasse im deutsch Kolonialreich, ed. Franz Bekker, 329–356. Stuttgart: Steiner Verlag, 2004.

Sauerteig, Lutz. "Die Deutsche Gesellschaft zur Bekämpfung der Geschlechtskrankheiten (DGBG), 1902–2002." *Aktuelle Dermatologie* 28 (2002): 393–397.

———. "Ethische Richtlinien, Patientenrechte und ärztliches Verhalten bei der Arzneimittelerprobung." *Medizin Historiches Journal* 35 (2000): 303–334.

———. "'The Fatherland is in Danger, Save the Fatherland!' Venereal Disease, Sexuality and Gender in Imperial and Weimar Germany." In *Sex, Sin and Suffering: Venereal Disease and European Society,* ed. Roger Davidson and Lesley Hall, 76–92. London: Routledge, 2001.

———. *Krankheit, Sexualität, Gesellschaft. Geschlechtskrankheiten und Gesundheitspolitik in Deutschland im 19. und früheren 20. Jahrhundert.* Stuttgart: Franz Steiner Verlag, 1999.

———. "Medizin und Moral in der Syphilisbekämpfung." *Medizin, Gesellschaft und Geschichte* 19 (2000): 55–70.

———. "Salvarsan und der 'ärztliche Polizeistaat': Syphilistherapie im Streit zwischen Ärzten, pharmazeutischer Industrie, Gesundheitsverwaltung und Naturheilverbänden (1910–1927)." In *Medizinische Bewegungen im Deutschen Reich (ca. 1870–ca. 1933),* ed. Martin Dinges, 161–200. Stuttgart: Franz Steiner Verlag, 1996.

———. "Sex Education in Germany from the Eighteenth to the Twentieth Century." In *Sexual Cultures: Themes in Sexuality,* ed. Franz Eder, Lesley Hall, and Gert Hekma, 9–33. Manchester: Manchester University Press, 1999.

Schmidt, Heike. "Colonial Intimacy: The Rechenberg Scandal and Homosexuality in German East Africa." *Journal of the History of Sexuality* 17, no. 1 (2008): 25–59.

Schneppen, Heinz. *Sansibar und die Deutschen: Ein besonderes Verhältnis 1844–1966.* Münster: Lit, 2003.

Schulte, Regina. *Sperrbezirke: Tugendhaftigkeit und Prostitution in der bürgerlichen Welt.* Frankfurt: Syndikat, 1979.

Schwarz, Thomas. "Die Kultivierung des kolonialen Behehrens—ein deutscher Sonderweg?" In *Kolonialismus als Kultur. Literature, Medien, Wissenschaft in der deutschen Gründerzeit des Fremden,* ed. Alexander Honald and Oliver Simons, 85–103. Tübingen: A. Francke, 2002.

Scott, James. *Seeing Like a State: How Certain Schemes to Improve the Human Condition Have Failed.* New Haven, CT: Yale University Press, 1998.

———. *Weapons of the Weak: Everyday Forms of Peasant Resistance.* New Haven, CT: Yale University Press, 1985.

Sebald, Peter. "Das deutsche 'Fußvolk' in Togo 1884–1914." In *Transformationen der europäischen Expansion vom 16. bis zum 20. Jahrhundert. 4. Jahrestagung des Schwerpunktprogrammes der Deutschen Forschungsgemeinschaft. Forschungen zur kognitiven Interaktion europäischen Gesellschaften,* ed. Andreas Eckert and Jürgen Müller, 171–178. Rehburg-Loccum: Evangelische Akademie Loccum, 1997.

———. "Kolonialregime und Mischlinge. Das Beispiel der deutschen Kolonie Togo 1884–1914." In *Rassendiskriminierung, Kolonialpolitik und ethnisch-nationale Identität. Referate des 2. Internationalen Kolonialgeschichtlichen Symposiums 1991 in Berlin,* ed. Wilfried Wagner, 108–118. Münster: Lit Verlag, 1992.

———. *Togo 1884–1914. Eine Geschichte der deutschen "Musterkolonie" auf der Grundlage amtlicher Quellen.* Berlin: Akademie Verlag, 1988.

———. "Togo 1884–1900." In *German Imperialism in Africa: From the Beginnings until the Second World War,* ed. Helmuth Stoecker, 83–93. London: C. Hurst & Company, 1986.

Setel, Philip. "Comparative Histories of Sexually Transmitted Diseases and HIV/AIDS in Africa: An Introduction." In *Histories of Sexually Transmitted Diseases and HIV/AIDS in Sub-Saharan Africa,* ed. Philip Setel, Milton Lewis, and Maryinez Lyons, 1–15. Westport, CT: Greenwood Press, 1999.

Shineberg, Dorothy. "The Sandalwood Trade in Melanesian Economics, 1841–65." In *Peoples of the Pacific: The History of Oceania to 1870,* ed. Paul D'Arcy, 359–376. Burlington, VT: Ashgate/Variorum, 2008.

Sigerist, Henry. *Civilization and Disease.* Ithaca, NY: Cornell University Press, 1945.

Sippel, Harald. "'Im Interesse des Deutschtums und der weißen Rasse': Behandlung und Rechtswirkungen von 'Mischehen' in den Kolonien Deutsch-Ostafrika und Deutsch-Südwestafrika." *Jahrbuch für afrikanisches Recht* 9 (1995): 123–157.

———. "Rechtspolitische Ansätze zur Vermeidung einer Mischlingsbevölkerung in Deutsch-Südwestafrika." In *Rassenmischehen—Mischlinge—Rassentrennung. Zur Politik der Rasse im deutschen Kolonialreich,* ed. Franz Becker, 138–164. Stuttgart: Steiner Verlag, 2004.

Sissons, D. C. S. "*Karayuki-san:* Japanese Prostitutes in Australia, 1887–1916—I." *Historical Studies* 17 (1977): 323–341.

Smith, Andrea. "Not an Indian Tradition: The Sexual Colonization of Native Peoples." *Hypatia* 18, no. 2 (2003): 70–85.

Smith, Woodruff. *The German Colonial Empire.* Chapel Hill: University of North Carolina Press, 1978.

———. "Colonialism and the Culture of Respectability." In *Germany's Colonial Pasts,* ed. Eric Ames, Marcia Klotz, and Lora Wildenthal, 3–20. Lincoln: University of Nebraska Press, 2005.

Spitz, Vivien. *Doctors from Hell: the Horrific Account of Nazi Experiments on Humans.* Boulder, CO: Sentient Publications, 2005.

Spongberg, Mary. *Feminizing Venereal Disease: The Body of the Prostitute in Nineteenth-Century Medical Discourse.* Washington Square: New York University Press, 1997.

Spree, Reinhard. "Kurpfuscherei—Bekämpfung und ihre sozialen Funktion während des 19. und zu Beginn des 20. Jahrhunderts." In *Medizinische Deutungsmacht im sozialen Wandel des 19. und frühen 20. Jahrhunderts,* ed. Alfons Labish and Reinhard Spree, 103–121. Bonn: Psychatrie-Verlag, 1989.

Stachura, Peter. "Social Policy and Social Welfare in Germany from the Mid-Nineteenth Century to the Present." In *Germany: A New Social and Economic History,* vol. 3, *Since 1800,* ed. Sheilagh Ogilvie and Richard Overy, 227–250. London: Arnold, 2003.

Steinmetz, George. *The Devil's Handwriting: Precoloniality and the German Colonial State in Qingdao, Samoa, and Southwest Africa.* Chicago: University of Chicago Press, 2007.

Stepan, Nancy. "Biological Degeneration: Races and Proper Places." In *Degeneration: The Dark Side of Progress,* ed. Edward Chamberlain and Sander Gilman, 97–120. New York: Columbia University Press, 1985.

Stoler, Ann. "Making Empire Respectable: The Politics of Race and Sexual Morality in 20th-Century Colonial Cultures." *American Ethnologist* 16 (1989): 634–660.

———. *Race and the Education of Desire: Foucault's History of Sexuality and the Colonial Order of Things.* Durham, NC: Duke University Press, 1997.

———. "Rethinking Colonial Categories: European Communities and the Boundaries of Rule." *Comparative Studies in Society and History* 31 (1989): 134–161.

Tashiro, Elke. *Die Waage des Venus: Venerologische Versuche am Menschen zwischen Fortschritt und Moral.* Husum: Matthiesen Verlag, 1991.

Tobin, Robert. "*Venus von Samoa.* Rasse und Sexualität im deutschen Südpazifik." In *Kolonialismus als Kultur: Literatur, Medien, Wissenschaft in der deutschen Gründerzeit des Fremden,* ed. Alexander Honold and Oliver Simons, 192–220. Tubingen: A. Francke Verlag, 2002.

Ulrich, Anita. "Ärzte und Sexualität—am Beispiel der Prostitution." In *Medizinische Deutungsmacht im sozialen Wandel des 19. und frühen 20. Jahrhunderts,* ed. Alfons Labish and Reinhard Spree, 223–235. Bonn: Psychatrie-Verlag, 1989.

van Laak, Dirk. "Kolonien als 'Laboratorien der Moderne'?" In *Das Kaiserreich transnational: Deutschland in der Welt 1871–1914,* ed. Sebastian Conrad and Jürgen Osterhammel, 257–279. Göttingen: Vandenhoeck & Ruprecht, 2004.

van Onselen, Charles. *Studies in the Social and Economic History of Witwatersrand 1886–1914,* vol. I: *New Babylon.* New York: Longman, 1982.

Vaughan, Megan. *Curing Their Ills: Colonial Power and African Illnesses.* Stanford, CA: Stanford University Press, 1991.

———. "Health and hegemony: Representation of disease and the creation of the colonial subject in Nyasaland." In *Contesting Colonial Hegemony: State and Society in Africa and India,* ed. Dagmar Engels and Shula Marks, 173–201. London: British Academic Press, 1994.

Vicinus, Martha. "Sexuality and Power: A Review of Current Work in the History of Sexuality." *Feminist Studies* 8 (1982): 132–156.

von Trotha, Trutz. *Koloniale Herrschaft: zur soziologischen Theorie der Staatsentstehung am Beispiel des "Schutzgebietes Togo."* Tübingen: J. C. B. Mohr, 1994.

Walgenbach, Katharina. "Rassenpolitik und Geschlecht in Deutsch-Südwestafrika (1907–1914)." In *Rassenmischehen—Mischlinge—Rassentrennung. Zur Politik der Rasse im deutschen Kolonialreich,* ed. Franz Becker, 165–183. Stuttgart: Steiner Verlag, 2004.

———. *"Die weisse Frau als Trägerin deutscher Kultur": Koloniale Diskurse über Geschlecht, "Rasse" und Klasse im Kaiserreich.* Frankfurt: Campus, 2005.

Walther, Daniel. *Creating Germans Abroad: Cultural Policies and National Identity in Namibia.* Athens: Ohio University Press, 2002.

———. "Gender Construction and Settler Colonialism in German Southwest Africa, 1894–1914." *The Historian* 66, no. 1 (2004): 1–18.

———. "Racializing Sex: Same-Sex Relations, German Colonial Authority, and Deutschtum." *Journal of the History of Sexuality* 17, no.1 (2008): 11–24.

———. "Sex, Race and Empire: White Male Sexuality and the 'Other' in Germany's Colonies, 1894–1914." *German Studies Review* 33, no. 1 (2010): 45–71.

Wareham, Evelyn. *Race and Realpolitik: The Politics of Colonisation in German Samoa.* Frankfurt: Peter Lang, 2002.

Watts, Sheldon. *Epidemics and History: Disease, Power and Imperialism.* New Haven, CT: Yale University Press, 1997.

Weindling, Paul. "Bourgeois values, doctors and the state: The professionalization of medicine in Germany 1848–1933." In *The German Bourgeoisie: Essays on the Social History of the German Middle Class from the Late Eighteenth to the Early Twentieth Century,* ed. David Blackbourn and Richard Evans, 198–223. London: Routledge, 1993.

———. *Health, Race and German Politics between National Unification and Nazism, 1870–1945.* Cambridge: Cambridge University Press, 1989.

———. "Hygienepolitik als sozialintegrative Strategie im späten Deutschen Kaiserreich." In *Medizinische Deutungsmacht im sozialen Wandel des 19. und frühen 20. Jahrhunderts,* ed. Alfons Labisch and Reinhard Spree, 37–55. Bonn: Psychatrie-Verlag, 1989.

White, Luise. *The Comforts of Home. Prostitution in Colonial Nairobi.* Chicago: University of Chicago Press, 1990.

Widmer, Alexandra. "The Effects of Elusive Knowledge: Census, Health Laws and Modern Inconsistently Modern Subjects in Early Colonial Vanuatu." *Journal of Legal Anthropology* 1, no. 1 (2008): 92–116.

Wildenthal, Lora. *German Women for Empire, 1884–1945.* Durham, NC: Duke University Press, 2001.

———. "Race, Gender, and Citizenship in the German Colonial Empire." In *Tensions of Empire: Colonial Cultures in a Bourgeois World,* ed. Frederick Cooper and Ann Stoler, 263–283. Berkeley: University of California Press, 1997.

Zimmerer, Jürgen. *Deutsche Herrschaft über Afrikaner. Staatlicher Machtanspruch und Wirklichkeit im kolonialen Namibia.* Münster: Lit, 2002.

Zimmerer, Jürgen, and Joachim Zeller, eds. *Genocide in German South-West Africa: the Colonial War (1904–1908) in Namibia and its Aftermath.* Monmouth, Wales: Merlin Press, 2008.

Zurstrassen, Bettina. "Die Steuerung und Kontrolle der kolonialen Verwaltung und ihrer Beamten am Beispiel des 'Schutzgebietes' Togo (1884–1914)." PhD dissertation, Universität der Bundeswehr, 2005.

Index

Monographs in German History

Volume 1
Osthandel and Ostpolitik: German Foreign Trade Policies in Eastern Europe from Bismarck to Adenauer
Robert Mark Spaulding

Volume 2
A Question of Priorities: Democratic Reform and Economic Recovery in Postwar Germany
Rebecca Boehling

Volume 3
From Recovery to Catastrophe: Municipal Stabilization and Political Crisis in Weimar Germany
Ben Lieberman

Volume 4
Nazism in Central Germany: The Brownshirts in 'Red' Saxony
Claus-Christian W. Szejnmann

Volume 5
Citizens and Aliens: Foreigners and the Law in Britain and the German States, 1789–1870
Andreas Fahrmeir

Volume 6
Poems in Steel: National Socialism and the Politics of Inventing from Weimar to Bonn
Kees Gispen

Volume 7
"Aryanisation" in Hamburg: The Economic Exclusion of Jews and the Confiscation of their Property in Nazi Germany
Frank Bajohr

Volume 8
The Politics of Education: Teachers and School Reform in Weimar Germany
Marjorie Lamberti

Volume 9
The Ambivalent Alliance: Konrad Adenauer, the CDU/CSU, and the West, 1949–1966
Ronald J. Granieri

Volume 10
The Price of Exclusion: Ethnicity, National Identity, and the Decline of German Liberalism, 1898–1933
Eric Kurlander

Volume 11
Recasting West German Elites: Higher Civil Servants, Business Leaders, and Physicians in Hesse between Nazism and Democracy, 1945–1955
Michael R. Hayse

Volume 12
The Creation of the Modern German Army: General Walther Reinhardt and the Weimar Republic, 1914–1930
William Mulligan

Volume 13
The Crisis of the German Left: The PDS, Stalinism and the Global Economy
Peter Thompson

Volume 14
"Conservative Revolutionaries": Protestant and Catholic Churches in Germany After Radical Political Change in the 1990s
Barbara Thériault

Volume 15
Modernizing Bavaria: The Politics of Franz Josef Strauss and the CSU, 1949–1969
Mark Milosch

Volume 16
Sex, Thugs and Rock 'N' Roll: Teenage Rebels in Cold-War East Germany
Mark Fenemore

Volume 17
Cultures of Abortion in Weimar Germany
Cornelie Usborne

Volume 18
Selling the Economic Miracle: Economic Reconstruction and Politics in West Germany, 1949–1957
Mark E. Spicka

Volume 19
Beyond Tradition and Modernity: Aby Warburg and the Public Policies of Art in Hamburg
Mark A. Russell

Volume 20
A Single Communal Faith? The German Right from Conservatism to National Socialism
Thomas Rohkrämer

Volume 21
Environmental Organizations in Modern Germany: Hardy Survivors in the Twentieth Century and Beyond
William T. Markham

Volume 22
Crime Stories: Criminalistic Fantasy and the Culture of Crisis in Weimar Germany
Todd Herzog

Volume 23
Liberal Imperialism in Germany: Expantionism and Nationalism, 1848–1884
Matthew P. Fitzpatrick

Volume 24
Bringing Culture to the Masses: Control, Compromise and Participation in the GDR
Esther von Richthofen

Volume 25
Banned in Berlin: Literary Censorship in Imperial Germany, 1871–1918
Gary D. Stark

Volume 26
After the 'Socialist Spring': Collectivisation and Economic Transformation in the GDR
George Last

Volume 27
Learning Democracy: Education Reform in West Germany, 1945–1965
Brian M. Puaca

Volume 28
Weimar Radicals: Nazis and Communists between Authenticity and Performance
Timothy S. Brown

Volume 29
The Political Economy of Germany under Chancellors Kohl and Schröder: Decline of the German Model?
Jeremy Leaman

Volume 30
The Surplus Woman: Unmarried in Imperial Germany, 1871–1918
Catherine L. Dollard

Volume 31
Optimizing the German Workforce: Labor Administration from Bismarck to the Economic Miracle
David Meskill

Volume 32
The Masculine Woman in Weimar Germany
Katie Sutton

Volume 33
State and Minorities in Communist East Germany
Mike Dennis and Norman LaPorte

Volume 34
Fragmented Fatherland: Immigration and Cold War Conflict in the Federal Republic of Germany, 1945–1980
Alexander Clarkson

Volume 35
Death in East Germany, 1945–1990
Felix Robin Schulz

Volume 36
Sex and Control: Venereal Disease, Colonial Physicians, and Indigenous Agency in German Colonialism, 1884–1914
Daniel J. Walther

www.ingramcontent.com/pod-product-compliance
Ingram Content Group UK Ltd.
Pitfield, Milton Keynes, MK11 3LW, UK
UKHW021839100926
8556IPUK00004B/433

9 781782 385912